"If you never have ~~~~~~ away' from Sue McRoberts' excellent memoir of her journey through postpartum depression. What I love is that she not only takes her reader to the bottom of the pit, but also shows us the light shining through at the top. Sue handles scripture with ease and her feelings with honesty. When the two come together, there is an amazing fusion that brings insight and help. If you want to understand or if you think you already do, you will be educated and ultimately encouraged by reading *The Lifter of My Head*."

Jan Silvious, Author and Speaker
Big Girls Don't Whine & Fool-proofing Your Life

"Babies are soft, cuddly and adorable…unless you're scared, confused and agitated. Then, they are not so precious to enjoy. I was surprised to learn that postpartum depression can begin before the baby is born and last for months. One woman's story about her walk through the dark corridors of PPD can shed light on what it is, who is affected, when to seek help, how to communicate it, and where your life can go with or without help. Read this book and allow Susan to assist you or a loved one through PPD with the confidence that a person can be understood, rescued and healed."

Dr. Thelma Wells, D.D., President and Founder of A Woman of God Ministries and the Daughters of Zion Leadership Mentoring Program, Speaker: Women of Faith Conferences, Author: *God Is Not Through With Me Yet!* And more www.thelmawells.com

"In *The Lifter of My Head*, Susan McRoberts demonstrates the ministry of proximity. Though she can't be there with you geographically, her story makes it clear that she has been there and is with you emotionally and spiritually. Susan's journey with postpartum depression is marked by authenticity, struggle, ambivalence and hope. Most importantly, she explains clearly how the Lifter of her head came alongside her and invited her into healing. He will do the same for you through Susan's story. I plan to give my clients a copy of *The Lifter of My Head*—those who struggle with postpartum depression, and those who seek to better understand the challenge."

Dr. Dan Rotach
Licensed Marriage and Family Therapist

"It is our tendency, as readers, to seek out stories that parallel our own—that give us a sense that someone else has been where we have been. Sue McRoberts' story, told with amazing candor, takes the reader to the depths of her own struggle and a place that will seem strangely familiar to those who have experienced depression. But this book offers much more than a compelling story with which to identify. Through education about mental health resources, the immense value of friendship and community, and the power and hope that can come only from God, Sue tells us what we can do. I trust you will find, as I did, a powerful testimony that is both inspirational and practical."

Keith TerHaar, LPC

"Sharing from the authority of her own battle through postpartum depression, Sue McRoberts candidly unveils the self-portrait of a survivor. With compelling honesty and stunning vulnerability, she draws the reader into the depths of a mind compromised by mental illness, a spirit crushed by the culture's indifference, and a heart cured by the healing power of Jesus Christ. If you see yourself within these pages, you will also see a way out."

Rebecca Ingram Powell
Author, *Baby Boot Camp*
Columnist, *ParentLife* magazine

"As King David once penned the promise, 'O Lifter of my head,' Sue McRoberts allows us to hear her heart's deepest cry. This highly personal, vulnerable view of postpartum depression gives insight and first hand testimony to the condition which many new moms are fearful to admit. Sue's words give relief, hope, confidence in faith, and credence to any new moms who need someone who truly understands. I applaud this brave and powerful work!"

Bonnie Keen
Author/Speaker/Singer

the *Lifter* of my head

how God sustained me during postpartum depression

the *Lifter* of my head

how God sustained me during postpartum depression

Sue McRoberts

TATE PUBLISHING & *Enterprises*

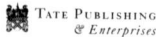 TATE PUBLISHING
& *Enterprises*

Tate Publishing is committed to excellence in the publishing industry. Our staff of highly trained professionals, including editors, graphic designers, and marketing personnel, work together to produce the very finest books available. The company reflects the philosophy established by the founders, based on Psalms 68:11,

"The Lord Gave The Word And Great Was The Company Of Those Who Published It."

If you would like further information, please contact us:
1.888.361.9473 | www.tatepublishing.com
Tate Publishing & *Enterprises*, LLC | 127 E. Trade Center Terrace
Mustang, Oklahoma 73064 USA

The Lifter of My Head
Copyright © 2007 by Sue McRoberts. All rights reserved.

No part of this publication may be reproduced, stored in a retrieval system or transmitted in any way by any means, electronic, mechanical, photocopy, recording or otherwise without the prior permission of the author except as provided by USA copyright law.

Scripture quotations marked "CEV" are from the Holy Bible; Contemporary English Version, Copyright © 1995, Barclay M. Newman, ed., American Bible Society. Used by permission. All rights reserved.

Scripture quotations marked "Msg" are taken from The Message, Copyright © 1993, 1994, 1995, 1996, 2000, 2001, 2002. Used by permission of NavPress Publishing Group. All rights reserved.

Scripture quotations marked "NIV" are taken from the Holy Bible, New International Version ®, Copyright © 1973, 1978, 1984 by International Bible Society. Used by permission of Zondervan Publishing House. All rights reserved.

Scripture quotations marked "NKJV" are taken from The New King James Version / Thomas Nelson Publishers, Nashville: Thomas Nelson Publishers. Copyright © 1982. Used by permission. All rights reserved.

Scripture quotations marked "NLT" are taken from the Holy Bible, New Living Translation, Copyright © 1996. Used by permission of Tyndale House Publishers, Inc. All rights reserved.

Scripture quotations marked "TAB" are taken from The Amplified Bible, Old Testament, Copyright © 1965, 1987 by the Zondervan Corporation and The Amplified New Testament, Copyright © 1958, 1987 by The Lockman Foundation. Used by permission. All rights reserved.

Scripture quotations marked "TEV" are taken from The Good News Bible: Today's English Version, New York: American Bible Society, Copyright © 1992. Used by permission. All rights reserved.

Scripture quotations marked "TLB" are taken from The Living Bible / Kenneth N. Taylor: Tyndale House, © Copyright 1997, 1971 by Tyndale House Publishers, Inc. Used by permission. All rights reserved.

Names, descriptions, entities and incidents included in the story are based on the lives of real people. However, several names have been changed to protect the identity of those characters.

The opinions expressed by the author are not necessarily those of Tate Publishing, LLC.

This book is designed to provide accurate and authoritative information with regard to the subject matter covered. This information is given with the understanding that neither the author nor Tate Publishing, LLC is engaged in rendering legal, professional advice. Since the details of your situation are fact dependent, you should additionally seek the services of a competent professional.

Book design copyright © 2007 by Tate Publishing, LLC. All rights reserved.
Cover design & interior design by Janae J. Glass

Published in the United States of America

ISBN: 978-1-6024731-3-3

07.02.05

"But You, O Lord, are a shield for me, my glory, and the lifter of my head."
(Psalm 3:3, TAB)

I dedicate this book to the women who have suffered. Let this be a new day!

"He put a new song in my mouth, a hymn of praise to our God!" (Psalm 40:3a, NIV)

Acknowledgments:

Numerous people played an important part in my healing. A special thanks goes to:

- Dr. Evan Friese, Darla, and Vicki. I believe you saved my life. Thank you for getting me the help I needed and most of all for calling me back that terrifying day.
- Barry for believing me and more importantly, understanding me. You made me see that postpartum depression wasn't a life sentence. You equipped me well for life after the psych ward.
- Ann Marie for showing me the love of Christ in the most surprising place. Thank you for making me see mental health professionals as helpers not punishers. God bless you for being so much like Jesus.
- George and Merle, my fellow inmates. Do you know what day it is? I will always cherish your support and kindness. I can't begin to express my gratitude to you.
- Mary. You know me better than anyone on the planet and you still think there's hope for me! You helped me heal very deep wounds. You restored my sanity, self-esteem, spirit, and purpose.

- Cindy my mentor, prayer warrior, and greatest cheerleader. You believed in me, and what God was doing, when not many others did.
- The breakfast club: Stacy, Denise, Paula, and Verity. Thanks for your prayers and for letting me go through it all without judgments or questions. You were there with me in the depths now let's celebrate at the heights!
- The ladies from my small group. You kept my sad self anchored in God's power through your prayers. I can't imagine how much harder this year would have been without you. You saw me come full circle. Praise God for the year we had together.
- Chrissy. Thanks for listening even way after I thought it was all over. When I was scared, you never left my side. I'm so blessed to have you as my friend.
- Mom, Aunt Carolyn, Marie, Kristin, and Jill. There wasn't a thing you could do but listen and you listened well! Thank you for letting me ramble and cry. Thank you for loving me when I was hurting.
- Pam. Thank you for your input on my earliest chapters and tolerating all my exclamation points.
- Patty. Thanks for your insight on the early chapters and for challenging me to the very end.
- Mike and Grace. I have been humbled by your generosity and belief in God's work in my life.
- Tate Publishing. You gave me a chance and again proved to me that God's mighty hand has been behind this from day one.

- My friends at Salem Baptist, Salem Avenue Baptist, and Peace Lutheran. Thanks for your encouragement along the journey. Carlyn and Tim, Lisa and Keith, Dan and Denise, God bless you for your compassion and kindness. To Salem's Stephens Ministry team, thanks for letting me tell my story for the first time.
- My hand-picked editorial staff made up of my husband, Stacy L., Paula, Stacy H., Patty and Cindy. You saved my hide and you know it. Thanks for your hard work and the countless hours you gave to my project. Cindy, thank you for helping me finish well.
- Brian. You were my rock when my whole world was sand. You came alongside me and made me laugh again. I can't believe what you endured. It's finally come time for us to close this chapter of our life.
- God: my savior, sustainer, counselor, strong tower, peace, help, shelter, foundation, defense, comforter, fortress, confidence, hope, the lifter of my head. I can't wait to see what you have in store.

Table of Contents

Foreword
19

In the Beginning
25

Pregnancy and Other Risk Factors
41

The Cliffs of Insanity
51

The 5th Floor
67

Post-Traumatic Stress
91

The Unquiet Mind
97

Friends God Gave Me
111

Healthcare Professionals God Used
133

The Lifter of My Head
145

Life After the Psych Ward
161

Foreword

Women with postpartum depression know something is not right. They know they are not feeling the feelings, saying the words, or doing the things that new mothers who feel good do. Women describe this in many ways, I just don't feel like myself or I've never felt like this or something's wrong, I just don't know what it is. They may seek help right away, they may deny that it's bad enough to get help, or they may sit tight doing nothing, secretly hoping it goes away by itself—but they all know something is terribly wrong.

Even today, after all we have learned about mental illness and childbirth and how vulnerable women are during this time, we continue to struggle with the juxtaposition: How can I want and love this baby so much and feel so bad? It's a struggle that keeps some women totally shut off from their world and compels others to search frantically for relief. Either way, they are lost somewhere between what they had hoped for and what they feared most.

When a mother holds her baby and wonders if she'll ever love him enough or be good enough to take care of him or whether he'd be better off without her, there is little comfort we as professionals can provide. We can say the right words, we can cite the right literature, and we can reassure her and offer the wisdom of our experiences. But when the dispirited woman sitting in our offices is haunted by despairing thoughts and believes in her heart that she has failed at the one thing she has spent her life yearning for, she needs more than words. She needs proof.

The women I treat in my practice often ask me if I had postpartum depression. I tell them I did not, aware that I am undoubtedly disappointing a number of them. That's because nothing can quite address the isolating anguish a new mother suffering from depression feels, like the words of another mother who has suffered and recovered. Women may certainly be relieved when they go to their doctors or start medication or begin therapy. But when they can hear or read the words of someone who has experienced a similar trauma, they begin to believe they might actually find healing. Sue McRoberts has written such a book. In *The Lifter of My Head: How God Sustained Me During Postpartum Depression*, McRoberts describes her personal ordeal with postpartum depression, never losing sight of her connection with her reader, bringing heartfelt compassion and experience to her words.

What she knows, only too well, is that many women who struggle with depression search for a power greater than themselves to help them through this unbelievably difficult time. All women, regardless of religious or spiritual beliefs, search for answers and meaning when they feel so out of control and fearful. McRoberts uses her life experience to enlighten others and pave the way for their recovery. She knows how hard it is to find help and eventually, well-being. She also knows how good it feels to finally get there.

She takes particular care in teaching the reader that self-care is an important part of healing, stating this in a line I have since quoted to several of my patients, "Saying no to others is more like saying yes to myself."

Indeed this is a book that Christian women will find helpful and tremendously supportive. But more importantly, this book illustrates how any religious faith can strengthen the spirit weakened by depression and serve as a guide throughout the lonely journey toward recovery.

Karen Kleiman, MSW
Founder & Director, The Postpartum Stress Center
and author of several books on postpartum
depression, including: *This Isn't What I Expected:
Overcoming Postpartum Depression* and *What am I
Thinking? Having a Baby After Postpartum Depression*

Introduction

I am not an expert in any field, nor do I have a medical background. I have only minimal textbook knowledge concerning psychology. I can't even begin to understand the human condition and the mind God gave us. I will not pretend to fully understand postpartum depression and its effects on women. I am writing this only to tell my story. I have heard it said that once you are an adult you can only be changed by the people you meet and the books you read. I hope and pray that by meeting me and God in these pages you will be changed. Maybe you need peace, comfort, or even strength. Maybe you need to see a light at the end of your dark tunnel. Maybe you love someone who needs these things. Maybe you're just curious. Surely God will give you what you need today. Thank you for reading my story. You are helping me heal.

"Write down for the coming generation what the Lord has done, so that people not yet born will praise him." (Psalm 102:18, TEV)

In the Beginning

> *"Let us then approach the throne of grace with confidence, so that we may receive mercy and find grace to help us in our time of need." (Hebrews 4:16, NIV)*

I don't know when the depression started. I don't recall when the anxiety hit. I do remember being discharged from the hospital with my baby, already feeling like something wasn't quite right. The nurse who discharged me asked, "Do you think you're getting depressed?" At the time I wanted to knock her out for even asking that question. How was I supposed to be feeling? Obviously, I felt terrible. I was bleeding like crazy, my milk had just come in, the baby pooped fifteen times a day, and I was going home to two strong-willed children. When I got home, I felt like a truck had run over my head a few dozen times. Breast-feeding the baby was excruciating at first. He nursed every two hours both day and night. However, I was so happy to see my baby boy. I walked the halls of the hospital for hours, pleading for him to come out. I was overwhelmed with joy when I finally got to see his face. Just touching him made me so happy. Immediately, I was deeply in love with him. It is difficult to express how one can be so ecstatic and in so much pain at the same time. Beyond my feelings of love for my son, I felt awful.

This first phase of postpartum depression is commonly known as the "baby blues." I despise that term. I've never met anyone that didn't feel overwhelmed and exhausted after giving birth. It is such an adjustment for the body, mind, and spirit. Your whole world is turned upside down, and you're supposed to instinctively know what to do with a helpless baby! I don't care if you've had one child or ten; it's a big transition at the very least. When people talk about "baby blues," it seems condescending, as if they could do it better. I have vowed to never ask anyone if they are having the "baby blues."

A few weeks after the baby was born, my husband asked me if I thought I was getting depressed. At least he didn't use the dreaded words! I was angry and embarrassed that he thought I wasn't adjusting perfectly to life with a newborn. I fought hard to not "get" postpartum depression. I truly believed I could will it all away. I assumed I was just sleep-deprived and struggling to juggle it all. I knew in my heart that life as we knew it would soon return. Then it happened—the baby started sleeping through the night.

There is this huge misconception that when the baby starts sleeping through the night you should too. As a result, you should start healing and feeling better. I knew that something was wrong when one of my friends asked me how I was feeling. I was doing terrible for no apparent reason. It dawned on me that I felt even worse than the day I gave birth! It made no sense to me that the baby was sleeping for eight or more hours, and I felt like death warmed over. It didn't matter what time of day it was; I felt depleted and downright sad. At 3:00 A.M. I felt the same as I did at 6:00 P.M. I had no sense of night and day. At night I could fall asleep, but I'd wake up several times. I could not go back to sleep no matter what I did. I would just lie there, waiting for morning to come. I didn't think about anything in those hours. I would just listen to the silent house. The silence brought me some sort of peace. Then, my insomnia took a turn for the worse.

It started with nightmares. I had multiple haunting dreams each night. I dreamed of people chasing and killing me. My dreams became terrifying and extremely violent. It felt like I was watching myself in a horror film. Next, I started having dreams about the baby. I kept seeing someone take him from me. I dreamed that I was holding him and taking a walk. It would seem so peaceful, and then someone would just rip him from my arms. I never saw the person who took the baby. He always wore a navy blue hooded sweatshirt and jeans. I never saw a face. I would float in and out of sleep, and I couldn't be sure when I was dreaming. Sometimes I was just thinking about things. But these things were bizarre, and I was so tired that I chalked it up to dreaming. I cannot begin to count the number of nights I woke up thinking I was pregnant. I would quickly realize I was just imagining things, but I still couldn't go back to sleep. I started dreaming about being pregnant. I would think all night about getting pregnant. There was no way that I could be pregnant, but I still obsessed about it. One day I had enough, so I called my obstetrician. Within the week I had extremely effective birth control, and my mind was at rest. I believed I would never worry about being pregnant again.

As a result of my sleepless nights, I started to physically struggle to get through the day. Tasks that were once routine became excruciating. It took all the strength I had to shower and get dressed. After that I was emotionally and physically done for the day. I usually felt like I needed a nap after my morning shower. Doing the breakfast dishes seemed like a monumental chore. More often than not, I would do the breakfast and lunch dishes minutes before my husband would arrive home in the evening. I would usually bawl the entire time. It seemed as painful as a root canal. Doing the laundry felt like torture. I would look at the piles of laundry and start to literally hyperventilate. I couldn't picture myself getting them washed, dried, folded, and put up. It would take me a week to get one load completely done, from the dirty basket to the closet. Hearing the phone ring would make me cry. I didn't have the strength to answer it. I didn't have the wherewithal to fake it well with everyone. The things that used to be just a normal part of the day were not normal any more. I could take care of my kids' basic needs but everything else was too much. I longed for my routine to normalize. I desperately wanted the chores of the day to be done without tears and pain.

Three main things were particularly difficult for me—all associated with memory. Making meals, personal hygiene and knowing where I was at all times were tall tasks. Not being able to make meals was the first thing that I noticed. Cooking meals was way out of my league. I've never been a great cook like my husband. I find no joy whatsoever in cooking dinner. I do it because we need to eat. I like trying new recipes but that's the extent of my cooking enthusiasm. At the depths of my depression, I just could not cook a meal. Getting all the ingredients together was nearly impossible. At least a dozen times I found myself in the middle of cooking only to discover that I didn't know how to finish. I couldn't remember how to make the meal.

The second thing was discovered in the bathroom. For a few weeks I couldn't remember if I'd washed my hair or not. I did a lot of washing, rinsing, and repeating. I often thought it was ridiculous that directions were printed on shampoo bottles. Now I believe that was probably suggested by a woman with postpartum depression! Once I caught myself in this wash, rinse, repeat cycle. I determined that I had to figure out a way to help myself. I would put shampoo in my hair to wash it, but I would only use one hand to rinse. That way, if I could still see the shampoo on my other hand, I could remember that I had washed my hair. I had to do this silly routine for a couple of weeks. I also forgot most days if I'd put on deodorant. I ended up putting on deodorant numerous times each day just to protect those around me!

The final thing I noticed was not so inconsequential. Multiple times a day I didn't know where I was. I could be standing, sitting, or driving, but I had no idea where I was. Time and time again I wouldn't remember where I was. Even after taking deep breaths and concentrating for a while, my mind would still come up blank. I would be changing the baby's diaper and not remember where the baby was. I was holding his diaper in one hand and his legs in the other, but I couldn't remember where he was! Dozens of times per day I would walk into a room to do something only to completely forget what it was. A few times I was holding a laundry basket full of clean clothes in my bedroom without a clue as to what I was doing with it. Hours later, I would be looking for the laundry. These chaotic days went on for weeks. At about six weeks postpartum it all came to a head.

At the time, I was helping lead my daughter's Brownie Girl Scout troop. My daughter and I were taking two girls to the meeting one night. The church where we met was only two miles away. Halfway there I became disoriented and panicky. I couldn't remember where I was going, how to get there, or why these people were with me. I had to pull the van over and pray that God would help me get to wherever it was that I was supposed to be going. God quieted me as only he can, and I found my way to the church. I mustered up enough strength to get out of the van and make it into the building. I knew instantly that my time was up with them. I realized I couldn't let them see me like this. The girls used to be so much fun, and so did I. I used to get so much energy by just being with them. They quickly became impossible to bear. My interest in them and my patience with them vanished almost immediately that night. Being with them was no longer an option. I believed that I could wish the negative feelings away. I felt inadequate as a mother, as a leader, as a mentor, and as a friend to my co-leaders.

The Lifter of My Head

For this last meeting with them, I was prepared with the Girl Scout lesson on paper but unprepared in my mind. It took me over a week to plan the 45-minute meeting. We were just starting in our new Brownie books, so there were lots of new and fun projects to discuss. The girls also got their new vests and patches. It should have been a really fun night, but it wasn't.

During the course of the meeting, I had my first round of racing thoughts. I felt like my brain was just frying. I recall that in middle school there was a commercial on television about drug use. They showed an egg and said, "This is your brain." Next, they showed a frying pan and the egg being fried. Then they shocked us by saying, "This is your brain on drugs." That's exactly how my brain seemed at that point. It didn't feel remotely like it was mine. To make it worse, I couldn't focus on anyone's face. I felt like I was looking through people. I couldn't read my lesson plans. It freaked me out that I couldn't read anything. Nothing made sense. I couldn't figure out if I was to read from the top or bottom or where. It seemed like I didn't even have my glasses on my face. The words were so jumbled that I experienced a type of blindness. All the words and voices and faces and lights ran together. I sensed people screaming at me. This was the first time I remember noise getting to me. (I used to teach school, everything from Kindergarten to high school, so I am no stranger to noise.) I've never experienced anything like this pain. It was as if every kid in the room was in my head screaming. I was irrationally irritated by their voices. The only thing worse than the noise level was the brightness of the lights. It was outrageous how much the light hurt my head. It was painful and disorienting. I remember not being able to breathe quite right. My air flow felt restricted. At the close of the meeting I started to hyperventilate. I got my daughter and left the building as quickly as I could.

Upon our arrival home, I fell apart. I yelled and cried with no explanation. I had so much negative emotion and energy, that it just sort of exploded out of me. It was that night that my three-year-old and six-year-old knew that I had lost it. After having my freak out session, it was time to get the kids ready for bed. Like all children, mine can tend to be difficult, and that behavior is not easy for someone suffering as I was. That night, my oldest child was in rare form. She finished brushing her teeth and started to wave her arms around and cry, because she couldn't find her Dixie cup of water that she needed to rinse out her mouth. I pointed to the cup and said, "Here's the cup." She started crying harder and said, "Which cup?" As she said this, over half of her toothpaste mess got all over her chin and pajamas. I then cupped my hands around the water cup and growled in a complete overreaction, "This cup!" My three-year-old laughed so hard he fell on the floor. My daughter decided it was pretty funny too. I think they thought I was trying to be funny. I don't remember feeling anything funny about that incident. I was crying uncontrollably and didn't know how I could get through the evening.

The very next morning I decided to do some research. I have a book titled *This Isn't What I Expected: Overcom-*

ing Postpartum Depression by Karen Kleiman and Valerie Raskin. I decided to flip through it and see what they had to say. I suffered from postpartum depression with my first child but needed a refresher course. As I started reading, I realized my symptoms were numerous and extreme. Kleiman and Raskin include a chapter on recognizing your postpartum depression. There are a few checklists that you can use to see if maybe you should call your doctor. There are some really basic statements like "I can't shake feeling depressed, no matter what I do. I cry at least once a day. I can't concentrate. I have no energy; I am tired all the time. It seems like I will feel like this forever." [1] I experienced everything on the first list I read. Then as I flipped through the book, I noticed a section I had skipped years before. It was about panic disorder with postpartum depression (PPD). I thought, *What on earth is that? I can't relate to that. They must be talking about truly crazy people!* Here are some of the "crazy" symptoms on the list: hot flashes, chills, trembling, nausea, inability to catch your breath, things feeling unreal, dizziness, numbness, feeling like you're having a heart attack. If I'd been using a highlighter, I would've colored the entire page yellow.

Next, I turned the page and discovered yet another "crazy" postpartum component: Obsessive-Compulsive Disorder (OCD). One of my favorite movies of all time is *What About Bob?* with Bill Murray and Richard Dreyfus. I thought that surely OCD could only manifest itself like it did with Bob. Bob is paralyzed with many fears. He has more phobias than one therapist can count. He can't touch door handles without holding a tissue that he uses as a barrier to the possible germs. I didn't have any Bob-like symptoms, so I thought for sure that this section couldn't describe me. I was wrong. My symptoms of OCD were quite different than the stereotype. Some people do worry incessantly about germs and counting things and cleaning and hand-washing. It wasn't until I did extensive reading that I realized that OCD can be very different than excessive cleanliness and exhaustive organizing. I had two main OCD symptoms.

First, I experienced repeated images that I initially believed to be real, but were not. I knew they were not normal, but I kept having them. It was as if someone was in my head planting bizarre thoughts. I didn't feel like I was really thinking these things. I felt very uncomfortable, guilt-ridden, and ashamed when I would have these weird things go through my head. I had terribly violent images. I saw the baby hurt over and over again in my dreams. Eventually these became nightmares during the day, but I was wide awake and seeing the same images as I did in my sleep. Sometimes I couldn't differentiate between my nightmares and my daytime thoughts. I felt just as asleep mentally during the day as I did during the night. I often imagined myself hurting the baby. Yet, I was so worried even about dropping him. I was terrified to walk across the house holding him. It was especially distressing for me to walk down the stairs with him. I would foresee myself falling and hurting him. Almost every time I walked down the stairs of our split-level home, I had to move methodically. A few times I pictured myself throwing the baby down. I never ever wanted to hurt the baby.

I never had any negative feelings toward him. I absolutely adored him with all my heart. These horrible images just overwhelmed and overtook me. I was scared that I was losing my mind.

The second OCD symptom that I suffered from was extreme doubt. After getting the boys in bed for naps, I would start working on whatever I felt like I could get done before they awoke. I would attempt to do some laundry or dishes. One day while ironing, I got this horrible feeling that my husband wasn't going to come home—ever. I couldn't shake the feeling of despair. I just couldn't imagine in a million years that he would want to come home. I would call him just to ask him when he would be coming home. I would call again in an hour or so to confirm the time. I was a wreck until he'd walk in the door. As soon as he walked in the house I was flooded with emotions. I was so happy he was there but so ashamed of myself. I just couldn't pull myself together. I couldn't take care of myself or the house. The kids were fed, bathed, dressed, and read to, but that's all I could manage. My boys were loved and played with every morning. My daughter and I would have special time together after school. We seemed to have fun as a family after dinner. On the surface life seemed normal. The kids were okay, and my husband hadn't picked up on my depression. But on the inside I was torn into bits. I was only a shell of myself. My spirit had been stomped on. My self-esteem was in the pits. My body image was shot. My confidence as a mother was shattered. I was convinced that my life was like the game Jenga. If one piece was moved, the whole tower of blocks

I called my life would collapse. I expected my husband to be the glue that kept us all together and happy. He never knew how scared I was. In my heart I really believed that one day he just wouldn't come home. I had nothing to contribute to the family but pain. I felt that I was no longer lovable.

Soon after I had my absurd concerns about my husband not coming home, I did some more research on PPD. I thought I would check out what was on the Internet. In my mind I had decided to call my OB, and I wanted to be well-prepared. I wanted to know exactly what I was attempting to describe to him. My symptoms were so many in number that I needed to see them in writing to remember them all. I found some checklists about feelings and whatnot, but they seemed rather vague. Those checklists were just not cutting it for me. Then I found the Mills Depression and Anxiety Symptom Feeling Checklist at the Postnatal Depression Support Association's website: www.pndsa.com. Basically, you are supposed to evaluate different feelings on a scale from 0–3. 0 means you never have the feeling, 1 means you have it from time to time, 2 means you have it quite often, and 3 means you have it most of the time. As I filled in the blanks with my numbers, I noticed a striking pattern: I was marking 3 on almost all of them. Out of forty items, I was suffering from thirty-three. There were only seven items that I hadn't experienced at all. The others I had experienced to the fullest. I don't recall my exact score on the test, but I knew it was off the charts. There was a key at the end of the checklist affirming that I had severe depression and anxiety and should contact a doctor. There were a few items that were alarming. If you experienced any of the symptoms highlighted in red, you were supposed to contact a doctor immediately. These shocking symptoms included fears or fantasies about hurting yourself, the baby or someone else; having scary thoughts; having weird or obsessive thinking; suicidal thinking; and preoccupation with death. I wasn't preoccupied with death, but I was experiencing the other scary symptoms. I took my checklist and decided to call the doctor.

I was able to see my obstetrician the next day. I tucked my checklist in my purse in case I got nervous and forgot to mention some things. I had already been to the obstetrician's office a few times postpartum so I was pretty tired of seeing these people. Nine months was long enough. When the nurse called my name I started to panic. I tried to pull myself together. I knew I needed help, but I didn't want anyone thinking I was a basket case. As we walked down the hall by the infamous scale, I about lost it. The nurse told me I didn't have to be weighed that day, and I just started bawling. The very idea of seeing that number on the digital display about made me vomit. I couldn't bear the bad news. At this point I'd only lost about fifteen pounds and was just irritated about it. My mood quickly changed. I became so angry with myself that I couldn't think straight. I was answering the nurse's questions, but I barely knew what she was asking. I was furious at myself for gaining so much weight during this pregnancy. It finally all made sense to me. I was suffering so badly from PPD because I was fat. At the time, it really made sense to me. I believed if I would just slim down, my life would normalize. Within the hour, I realized that those thoughts were irrational. I had no doubt that it was far more complex.

The nurse took my blood pressure, asked me a few questions, and left me with a sheet of paper. My eyes burned with tears as I attempted to fill out the worksheet for the doctor. It was a bare-bones screening for postpartum depression. There were only ten statements. I was supposed to rate my feelings over the last few weeks on a scale of one to ten. I feel sad. Sure, that was a ten. I cry for no reason. Again I marked ten. I comprehended that this assessment was not going to scratch the surface of my problems. For some really bizarre reason, I tried to suck it up and act like only those ten things were wrong. I forgot all about the paper I was carrying in my purse. I wanted to forget about all the really bad stuff. I thought the doctor might think I was a total lunatic. As a defense mechanism, I honestly forgot about the paper until I got home. The doctor prescribed me a small dose of antidepressant and off I went. He confirmed that I did indeed have PPD. I felt more alone than ever. I'd been given a chance to get help, and I had minimized my problems. I was angry with myself and scared at the same time. I knew that I had more than a textbook case of postpartum depression. I truly sensed that there was a lot more to come. I predicted that I would be back to see my obstetrician when I had the courage. Unfortunately, I fell apart before that happened.

Food for thought:

"Have you learned how to let Christ minister to you? Let me make this assignment: let Christ love you today. Curl up in His arms and tell Him you need Him. Until you learn to let Him serve you at the point of your need, you will never be truly free to serve others."[2]

—Beth Moore,
A Woman's Heart: God's Dwelling Place

Pregnancy and Other Risk Factors

"Jesus looked at them and said, 'With man this is impossible, but with God all things are possible.'" (Matthew 19:26, NIV)

My experience has been that at times, pregnancy felt impossible. It seemed to last forever. Neither rest nor comfort could be found. While using my own strength, pregnancy seemed daunting and cumbersome. However, with God all things are possible. Pregnancy can be bearable and enjoyable, even a worthwhile exercise in patience. Can I get an amen? Jesus meant that we could go through something like pregnancy and childbirth with him? God goes through something that intensely personal with us? That is awesome and humbling for me! Wouldn't those nine months go so differently if we leaned on God's strength? Wouldn't the birth process be less miserable? It is incredible to think that God is with us. I can tell you for a fact that he was with me during my pregnancy, labor, and delivery. If you have not previously included God in this process, you are really missing out on enormous blessings. I know I left him out of my first two pregnancies. With my first pregnancy, I never even gave God much thought. It never dawned on me that he cared about my pregnancy, emotions, or body. I knew he would protect the baby, and that's all I ever prayed for. With my second pregnancy, I was working and miserable. I was in a rut of feeling awful about being pregnant. I just wanted it to be over. That was my main focus. I remember being happy about having another baby, but that was it. I was a very unhappy pregnant woman. I threw a pity party more often than not. With my third pregnancy, things were completely different. I went into it fit and determined to stay that way. When I say fit, I mean completely fit: my weight, my emotions, my mind, my walk with God, my family life. Everything seemed to be so great in my life. The addition to our family could bring nothing but more happiness and fulfillment. I was staying home with my older children at the time, so there was no additional stress of day care or job responsibilities. It appeared like we had the life most people dreamed of. We went camping and swimming. We played sports in the yard. We went on bike rides. I continued to go to fitness classes. I felt like a million bucks for about six months. Then, the dreaded third trimester came, and my happy face was stripped from me.

At the beginning of my third trimester, I sprained my ankle. That injury crippled me. With fifteen or more extra pounds to lug around, crutches were unbearable. Taking care of my other two children became an even bigger chore. They spent most of my third trimester entertaining themselves. I spent weeks upon weeks icing my ankle, visiting doctors, and lying on the couch in tears. I was in so much pain that I found it difficult to sleep. I was exhausted but couldn't get comfortable enough to rest. As I tried different wraps, casts, boots, you name it—I gained weight. Gaining weight while trying to heal didn't help one bit. It made the whole process of hauling around a bum foot completely ridiculous. With three or four weeks until the arrival of the baby, I started to make a turnaround. I could walk and not feel too much pain. But the weight remained and reeked havoc on my body. I had never gained so much weight before. It made me more tired than I should have been. Just walking, sleeping, bathing, and things of that nature were cumbersome. I'm hesitant to admit it, but the last month was a nightmare for me. I'm not near as tough as I once bragged. As the physical part of pregnancy dragged me down, I started to become emotionally challenged. I detest when women speak loosely of the effects of hormones, so I don't say this lightly: my hormones were going berserk. As my body geared up for the coming of our child, my emotional health suffered. I could no longer keep my emotions in check. I cried and yelled over everything and nothing. I was a mess of emotions.

The last weeks were challenging, especially because I'd never gone into labor naturally before. With my first two babies, labor was induced. With my first baby, labor was induced due to extremely high blood pressure. With my second baby, my obstetrician just wanted to schedule it so he wouldn't miss an important golf date. With my third baby, I went into labor on my own. I had approximately four weeks to go in my pregnancy when I first thought I might be in labor. I went to the hospital, was examined, and sent home after a few hours to follow all of their out-patient directions. After arriving home, I understood that the end of this pregnancy was going to be different. I knew this would be the toughest one to endure. About ten days later, I returned to the hospital. I was embarrassed enough the first time. I waited for hours, made numerous phone calls, read all my baby books, and said many prayers before heading back to the labor and delivery floor. I was convinced I was in labor and that my water had broken. With a first baby, I could see how you might not know how to tell that your water has broken. With a third baby, there is no confusion. I knew my water was leaking. After keeping me for several hours, my contractions again ceased, and I was sent home. I was no longer embarrassed; I was humiliated. I can't begin to count how many people at the hospital asked me if this was my first baby. I was so irritated, I even became angry. I knew I was in labor. What I couldn't figure out was why the baby wasn't ready. I totally surrendered my anger and humiliation to God. I had a suspicion that God wasn't done with the baby just yet. Maybe his toenails weren't just right. Maybe his fingers needed more nurturing. Perhaps his precious lungs needed a little more time to strengthen. I had a certain calmness concerning the baby's arrival. Then it happened. My contractions started again.

Thirteen days before my due date, I started my last bout with labor. I woke up in the middle of the night with contractions. I couldn't breathe for the longest time. Eventually the contractions waned, and I rested. The next morning after breakfast, the contractions started up again. After rapidly reaching regular and lengthy contractions, I started doubting myself. There was no way I was even going to call a nurse, let alone show up at the hospital again. As my contractions became more painful, I couldn't even walk, talk, or think. I remained confident that the labor would again subside. When the level of pain became evident to my husband, he insisted I at least call a nurse at the hospital. After a few hours, my contractions had not subsided. I made babysitting arrangements for the children and headed to the hospital. I told the nurse on the phone that I would not go to the hospital and leave without a baby. I was on a mission! After a long day and night of contractions stopping and starting, I reached the point of no return. They moved me to the labor and delivery room, out of triage. I'm not joking when I share with you that my labor again stopped. I was dilated to seven centimeters when my body just stopped. In a strange way, I was disappointed when they decided to jump start my labor with medication. I had experienced so much to that point that I just wanted to prove that I could do it. I didn't want medicine, but I did want a baby. I held my stomach in a different manner in those last hours. I wanted to see my baby. I didn't care how it happened; I was ready. The last hours were tough. I was exhausted and emotional. The experience consumed my energy and left me feeling half dead. Having strangers exclaim to me, "It's a boy!" temporarily wiped out the pain. Holding him made me feel so proud and fulfilled. We had survived a difficult journey together. Everything about him was perfect; I knew God's timing was just right.

Why do I want you to know about my difficult labor and delivery? In my humble opinion, the difficulty of my last trimester, especially the last month, was a catalyst for my postpartum depression. I know that it put me at a huge risk. My first labor and delivery was a nightmare and I had postpartum depression. My second pregnancy, labor, and delivery were all a breeze. I felt great after giving birth the second time. My third experience was physically and emotionally difficult and again, I had postpartum depression. You will be hard-pressed to read about this anywhere else. I've searched high and low for information on this topic. I can't find any medical evidence or documentation that this has been true for anyone else. But I see a clear pattern in my own experiences. I believe that my rough times with pregnancy and birth were some of the most significant risk factors for my postpartum depression.

What else can cause postpartum depression? Most experts agree that postpartum depression isn't caused by any one thing in particular. Obviously, giving birth is the one common denominator. There are multiple factors that can potentially make you vulnerable to such depression. According to www.pregnancytoday.com, most experts agree that, "it [PPD] involves a combination of hormonal, psychosocial, and environmental influences." Many things can put a woman at risk for PPD. According to Pregnancy Today some of them are:

- previous PPD
- family history of anxiety or depression (genetic predisposition)
- unplanned pregnancy
- unsupportive spouse

- recent separation or divorce
- major loss in past two years (death of loved one, for example)
- obstetric complications
- environmental stressors 1

Some women can have these risk factors and never develop full-blown depression. The list of factors can only increase your susceptibility to the illness. According to www.postpartumstress.com, there are even more risk factors. These are all part of a PPD risk assessment to be used during pregnancy. If any of these apply to you then you should discuss them with a doctor before you give birth:

- I was not happy to learn I was pregnant.
- My partner was not happy to learn I was pregnant.
- I have had a previous episode of postpartum depression and/or anxiety successfully treated with therapy and/or medication.
- I might have experienced symptoms of postpartum depression following previous births, but I never sought professional help.
- I have had one or more pregnancy losses.
- I have a history of depression/anxiety that was not related to childbirth.
- I have lost a child.
- I have been a victim of the following:
    -Childhood sexual abuse
    -Childhood physical abuse

-Physical assault by someone you know
  -Physical assault by a stranger
  -Physical assault during this pregnancy
  -Sexual assault by someone you know
  -Sexual assault by a stranger
- There is a family history of depression/anxiety, treated or untreated.
- I have a history of severe PMS.
- I have experienced suicidal thoughts or have considered doing something to hurt myself in the past.
- I do not have a strong support system to help me if I need it.
- I have a history of drug or alcohol abuse.
- People have told me I'm a perfectionist.
- During this pregnancy, I have experienced some emotions about which I am very concerned.
- I feel sad.
- My relationship with my partner is not as strong as I'd like it to be.
- I am not likely to admit when I need help.
- During the past year, I have experienced an unusual amount of stress. (a move, job loss, divorce, loss of loved one)
- I have little interest in things that I used to find pleasurable.
- I am having anxiety attacks.
- I am more irritable and/or angry than usual.
- I just don't like myself.
- Sometimes, I feel like I can't shake off these bad feelings no matter what I do.

- I'm afraid if I tell someone how I really feel, they will not understand or they will think something is really wrong with me.[2]

Some women don't have many of these risk factors, but can suffer horribly with depression. If you or someone you know has any of these risk factors, they should not be taken lightly. I had several of the risk factors and never knew they were significant until I did extensive research. It is my hope and prayer that more women will know, going into motherhood, what to expect. If you know what could happen, you had better alert the people in your support system. You can access all the resources available to you. You must start reading appropriate literature. You should discuss concerns with your obstetrician, spouse, and friends. The more you know, the better prepared you will be.

You shouldn't go into motherhood naively. You may have several risk factors for postpartum depression. No one ever told me about PPD when I was pregnant for the first time. I'm telling you, so that *you* can be proactive. You can take charge of your health—emotionally, physically, mentally, and socially. God expects us to take good care of ourselves. Unfortunately, life happens and we aren't always ready for what might hit us. That doesn't mean we can't learn and grow from our experiences. I now know what to expect. I desperately long for you to be prepared. I don't want anyone to have the truck of PPD run over them like it did me. Get ready. God bless you if you never experience PPD. Hopefully, you can help spread the word, so more women are prepared for what could happen. One thing I've learned: if God blesses our family with another baby, I'm ready. I'm not thrilled about the prospect, but I know that God would see me through it all over again. I'm now better prepared and not as scared to seek help. I'm not timid about asking others to pray for me. I've got a stronger will to live life well. Postpartum depression didn't get the best of me. Instead, I feel like I got to see the best of God. I saw more of God because I sought him as never before. He revealed himself to me in some dire situations. My circumstances took everything out of me. But I had just a little faith in a big God who gave me everything I needed. I asked for immediate help; he provided it. I asked for support; he gave it. I asked for his power; he showed it. I asked for peace; he gave it. I asked him to stick it out with me; he did. I asked him to protect my family; he did. I asked to be healed; he did it. With God all things *are* possible.

Food for thought:

"We are not human beings on a spiritual journey. We are spiritual beings on a human journey."

—Dr. Stephen Covey, author and speaker

The Cliffs of Insanity

"My tears have been my food day and night. Why are you so downcast, O my soul? Why so disturbed within me? Put your hope in God, for I will yet praise him, my Savior and my God." (Psalm 42:3; 5–6, NIV)

As time passed, I still struggled with the fear of becoming pregnant. One particular time I thought about it, I believed with all my heart I was. It was perhaps the most bizarre experience of my life. When I awoke that morning, my first thought was of being pregnant. I quickly became hysterical and just couldn't believe this was happening to me. I tried to pull myself together for the kids' sake. It was time for our morning routine to begin. We had to eat breakfast, brush teeth, pack lunches, get dressed, check backpacks, etc. The kids didn't have time for me to freak out about being "pregnant." Nevertheless, it was a typical day for the kids. I took my daughter and her neighbor friend to elementary school without a hitch. I then took my son to preschool. He was so thrilled to be at school that day. They were having a popcorn and movie day. I'll not soon forget how happy he was that morning. Back at the house, his mommy was a wreck.

When the baby and I arrived home, one of my girlfriends called. I wanted so badly to hear her voice, but

I was scared I wouldn't be able to keep up the charade of being happy and feeling great. She called to check on me, which I found really strange. I couldn't remember the last time anyone had checked on me. It bothered me that someone could tell something was wrong. The previous night had been a girls' night out with some ladies from church. When I didn't go without contacting anyone, my friend saw that as a red flag. I opened up a little bit about what I was experiencing. She was very supportive, but I wasn't totally honest. I quickly explained that I just wasn't feeling good. How can one sugarcoat postpartum depression? I could, and I became very good at it. I don't remember all that we discussed, but I know that I hung up as quickly as I could. I felt like the dam was about to burst.

After our conversation, I fed the baby and put him down for a nap. One of my favorite things to do in those early postpartum weeks was to take a hot bubble bath. A bath was definitely in order that morning. Something about the quietness of that time is unforgettable to me. It was the calm before the storm. Just a few minutes into the bath, I started trembling, panicking about being pregnant again. My hysteria was short-lived, but only because my frenzied state promptly turned delusional. I realized that I wasn't pregnant after all because I had experienced a miscarriage. I was distraught as I mourned my miscarriage—one that I never had. As swiftly as I became irrational about being pregnant, I became psychotic when I grieved over my imagined miscarriage. As I shook in the tub, my delusion deepened. I began rubbing my stomach, my empty womb, and talked to the dead baby. I even called her by name. I recall telling her how much I wanted to see her. For that thirty-minute period I believed with all my heart and mind that I had experienced pregnancy and loss. I knew I'd never hold my baby girl. I felt guilt for losing her. I was convinced that I had done something terribly wrong, or I would still have her growing inside me. I then heard my newborn squeak in his bedroom. Just that simple noise brought me back to reality, and I was cognizant of my delusional condition.

It was intimidating to feel like my mind was no longer mine. I felt like I had no control over my own thoughts. I felt nauseated and light-headed. As I let the water out of the tub, I felt sweaty and weak. I doubted I could stand. My mind raced as the room spun. It almost seemed like I was hallucinating. The world no longer appeared real. The lights became ultra illuminated. I wanted to scream because the lights hurt so much. Closing my eyes didn't bring any relief. I wanted out of the pain. I hyperventilated as I searched for an answer. I had my first official panic attack. I was frightened by what my body and mind experienced. I wanted to go to sleep so it would just stop. I was convinced that if I slept for a week I'd wake up okay. Couldn't I just sleep all this away? I remembered that I had painkillers in the cabinet that my doctor prescribed after I had the baby. That medicine made me feel awful, but with it I could sleep through a tornado. I thought if I took the rest of the bottle I could sleep for a week or more. I never wanted to die. I just knew the pills would ease my pain, alter my state of mind. I just wanted the crisis to pass. Then I concluded that painkillers mixed with the anti-depressant that I was already taking would most likely harm me. So I spent some time thinking about drowning myself in the tub. I guessed that would be painless. But I assumed that would really be scary, and I might actually die. It became clear to me that was a stupid idea. Besides, one of my biggest fears is dying by drowning. In college I read *The Awakening* by Kate Chopin. In the book, an unhappy wife and mother kills herself by walking out into the ocean without returning. I always thought she was a coward. I detested reading that book, but I am so thankful I did. The vivid ocean scene in my mind forced me to reconsider my thoughts. Rapidly, my delusions and hallucinations curtailed. My suicidal thoughts subsided.

The only way in which I can account for what happened was that my brain short-circuited. (Later my psychologist would concur with me.) I am not a scientist, but I am convinced that is precisely what occurred. I was in the middle of a neurological and biological emergency. It's as if something fried in my brain for a short while. I was at the climax of my crisis which had been escalating for weeks. Conceivably, it was all my mind could take and I collapsed, both emotionally and physically. I am thankful to God to this day that one small part of my brain was still functioning on all cylinders. I knew I was in crisis mode and needed to seek help immediately. I was aware that I was out of control. All I could think of was to call my obstetrician. I knew that if I could talk to him he could help me. I had no preconceived notions as to what he would offer. But, I was strongly convinced that he could make everything right.

I was rattled to my core as I got dressed. As I brushed my hair I pictured someone hurting the baby. I don't honestly know who was hurting the baby. Numerous people asked me if I thought about hurting the baby, but I don't think I ever did. The thoughts didn't feel like mine. I repeatedly saw someone throwing him. As I brushed my teeth, I kept picturing myself attempting to catch and save the baby. Time and time again I would fail to save him. These thoughts were so real. With all of these serious symptoms hitting me at once, I knew I was in grave trouble.

In my desperation I made the phone call that would save my life. As I spoke to the receptionist on the phone, I tried to make my voice sound put together and calm. I wanted to scream into the phone for help, but I couldn't. I wanted someone to physically come to my house and rescue me. Naturally my obstetrician was booked for the day. All the other doctors were booked that day too. There weren't any physician's assistants available either. I've never called that office and not been able to see someone. The woman on the phone suggested I see someone in family practice. I politely replied that that was not a good idea. I knew at that point that I needed more than an office visit. Fortunately, God knew that ahead of time. I believe he orchestrated the whole scenario. He made it impossible for me to make an office visit so that I would seek the appropriate help. I plainly explained my situation to the receptionist, and she promptly transferred me to triage. The triage nurse was busy and the receptionist came back on the line. She took my name and number and promised the triage nurse would return my call as soon as humanly possible. I clung to the phone and to the hope of someone's voice. The phone did indeed ring. I was hesitant to answer the phone, because I felt that in a few moments I would fall apart. Darla was the triage nurse who called me back. I remembered her voice from a previous appointment. She was the nurse who did my prenatal nutrition visit at three months. I could picture her face and it was instantly comforting. Darla gave me permission to fall apart. She didn't have to ask many questions. She knew what she was hearing was critical. It was amazing how well she could read me. I believe that God gave her special listening ears that day. She informed me that I needed to call my husband and get to the emergency room. Unfortunately, my husband had no idea what was going on. He knew I was depressed, but we rarely discussed it. He had no clue as to the depth of my pain. I had hidden such pain from him before, and I hoped I could do it again. Thank God Darla knew what was racing through my sick head. She sensed that I wouldn't call my husband for help. She asked if she could contact him for me. I felt like someone lifted a mountain of fear off of my shoulder. It was okay with me that Darla told my husband since I couldn't muster the strength to do it myself. I was ashamed, embarrassed, and filled with guilt. I didn't want my husband to think I was stupid. To be honest, at that point I felt stupid. While I was getting ready for my husband to come get me, Darla was desperately trying to reach him at work. He was in the middle of a presentation when someone from security contacted him. The only message he received was that there was an emergency at home. Naturally he thought the house was on fire or something happened with one of the kids. He had no idea that it was something much worse. At that time there wasn't much physical deterioration to see but the emotional and psychological damage was mounting.

My husband arrived, and we left to pick up our son from preschool. It broke our son's heart to leave his special movie day at school, but he was soon content to know that he would be playing at a neighbor's house for the remainder of the day. We made arrangements for our daughter to be picked up from school. My friend picked her up and then took both of the kids for burgers and ice cream. Later my daughter couldn't wait to share with me that my son only ate ice cream for dinner. The poor little guy was stressed out so I was fine with his dinner choice. God bless him for eating anything that day! Once the kids were settled, we could focus on getting me some help. I was under the impression that a counselor and a psychiatrist would meet me at the emergency room. We arrived at the ER and went through the tedious process of checking in. I have been to the ER for concussions and badly sprained ankles, but I assumed this experience would be significantly different. The check-in process was the same—height, weight, blood pressure, temperature. Next began the barrage of staff—nurses, doctors, and students.

I can't recall all of the people I saw in those first hours at the hospital. They all run together in my memory. I saw a doctor who needed to make sure I wasn't physically ill. I saw a handful of nurses who didn't do anything at all.

In retrospect I think they were just keeping tabs on me, recording my behaviors and moods. Eventually a needs assessment staff member arrived. This was the beginning of the help I so desperately needed. She had a handy dandy laptop full of personal questions that had to be answered. My husband was escorted out, and I was to bare all. We discussed everything from all three of my pregnancies, my family history, my childhood, my adulthood, my education, my children, my marriage, and most of all my current mental health. I have no idea how long I answered questions, but it seemed like days. I had been holding so much in for so many months—to be honest, years—that it was as if someone finally allowed me to unload. In about forty-five minutes I debriefed a stranger on my entire life story. In a nutshell, on paper, my life looked pretty sad indeed. I became more depressed as I heard my own stories come out of my mouth. I couldn't believe all that I had endured over a lifetime, and no one ever suggested to me that I should seek professional help. It was time.

I reflect back on these early hours of my insanity and I picture cliffs. In one of my favorite movies, *The Princess Bride*, this obnoxious Sicilian guy yells from his boat, "The cliffs of insanity!" I don't have a clue as to what he was talking about or why he was so passionate about the cliffs, but it's one of the best parts of the movie. Could a very funny movie provide me with the title for my very serious book? I fell in love with the idea. I could picture the guy from *The Princess Bride*, and it brought me some much needed levity. Apparently many people associate cliffs with insanity. As I did some research I ran across a book entitled *Cliffs of Despair: A Journey to the Edge*. Reading some of the book, I realized that it was about suicide. Nearly five hundred people have died at Beachy Head, a four mile long cliff on the south coast of England. Almost all of those deaths have been suicides. This haunting place is the third most popular suicide spot on the planet. Knowing only that much about the book, I gave up my idea for my book title. I could laugh at my own thoughts, but I didn't want the book to scare people to death.

The cliffs symbolize two things for me. First, they represent death. Falling off, jumping off, driving off...all these things imply death. In college I had a geography professor that pleaded with us to drive along the coastal highway in California. He promised it would be an experience we'd never forget. For years I dreamed of driving on Highway 1. For our ten-year wedding anniversary, my husband and I took a weekend trip to San Francisco. We rented a snazzy convertible and drove for hours on Highway 1. I even took snapshots of the highway signs so I could remember the day. All those years of fantasizing about the drive were wasted. I was terrified while my husband drove. It was like being on an endless roller coaster. If he had sneezed just once, we would have died. It was breathtaking, but not in a pleasant way. Cliffs truly represent fear, car sickness, tension, and death for me. I did go through a very intense, yet short-lived, desire to die. I don't want to pretend that I didn't. Never in my life have I understood what suicidal people must be thinking. I've always judged them and never had much sympathy. It wasn't until I experienced real pain and genuine insanity that I reached the point of empathy. I don't believe that I wanted to die, I just didn't know how else to end the pain. I was so frightened by my thoughts, emotions, actions, feelings, and pain. I felt so alone and unique, like no one had ever been through this before me. My suicidal thoughts were brief, but the cliffs of insanity remained.

Secondly, the cliffs depict walls. My depression, anxiety, and insanity were like massive walls in my daily life. I couldn't get to the other side of the walls to where my real life was. I was stuck in the mud and rocks of my physiological mess. I longed to find the strength to knock down the walls. I tried climbing them, but I just kept falling, and the harder I tried the harder I fell. I desperately believed I could will this all away. I was convinced that I had done something wrong to make this happen. I became engulfed in my negative thinking patterns. I had distorted self-perceptions. I criticized myself day and night. In the middle of the night I would lie awake and think of all I had done wrong that day. I couldn't get a handle on things. I couldn't figure out how to keep the house clean, do the laundry, make three meals a day, get the kids to school, take care of the baby, and smile all in the same day. I didn't feel like I could do anything right. Here is a summary of what would go through my mind during a given day.

> I can't believe it's time to get up. Didn't I just feed the baby? Did yesterday ever end? Is it really a new day? There's so much to do. The floor needs to be mopped. The diaper pail is full to the brim again. The dog needs to be fed. Had I run the vacuum in a week? I'm so sick of every day being so hard.

The baby only has five diapers left. The bills need to be paid. Had I read my Bible since the baby was born? I've got to get control of my emotions. I have at least three friends in crisis who need me. What day is it? We desperately need groceries. I really need to use the bathroom. Maybe I can go in a few minutes. My OB thinks I am stupid. My husband has to know that I haven't ironed in three months. The bathroom looks like animals use it. The rest of the house looks like animals live in it. Had I called my sick aunt? I forgot to return a phone call from the volunteer coordinator at the elementary school. I haven't accomplished anything worthwhile today. I think my son's preschool teacher hates me. Why aren't my anti-depressants working yet? God, are you there? Why won't you make it better? What did I do wrong? I think I'm a good mother. Why do I feel like such a bad mother? I don't feel like myself at all. I wish I could just laugh and quit crying. I'm so tired I feel like I could die. This is the worst day of my life. Do we have bread? Am I ready to sing on the praise team at church yet? Why haven't I been going to Bible Study on Wednesday nights? No one feels this lousy after having a baby. I hadn't cleaned out the junk drawer in the kitchen for weeks. The garage is a disaster. I wish I could have a Milky Way and some French fries. I am so stupid. The baby nurses every two hours, and I'm sick of it. My husband thinks I'm stupid, I can tell by the way he looks at me. I have twenty e-mails in my inbox and I don't care. I don't want to talk about Girl Scouts or how I'm doing or when are we going to have a play date. Did I get the mail yet? I guess I should do the dishes while it's quiet. The baby's awake again! Boy, do I look fat. I love my kids, but I hate being home all the time. Yes, he's sleeping through the night! Why do I feel so tired then? I wish I had a real job. My husband would be so much happier with someone else. My kids must know I'm crazy. They are going to need therapy. I wish I could just relax. I should make some cookies for the kids. We're out of eggs. Did I put the laundry in the dryer? I need to call my mother. I forgot to call the pediatrician and make an appointment. The trash needs to go out before the trash man gets here. Does recycling go out this week? There he goes, driving down the street. I can't believe I missed him. Have I brushed my hair today? I really should catch up on some reading. I don't know if the baby's developing correctly unless I read the book the nurse gave me when I was discharged. I've got to spend some time reading up on that. What about my depression? I've got to read some more on that. I think I'm getting depressed. We've got brunch this morning at church. I guess I'll have to get donuts again. I keep forgetting to make something to take. I guess I should do the dishes from last night before my daughter gets home from school. I wonder if people can tell that I've been crying all day. Can they tell I want to explode? Do people notice my fun new tics? I can't stop scratching my face. My hands itch too. My face must be swelling. I'm going to have a heart attack. What day is it? I don't think I've used the bathroom yet today. The baby's awake again. Have the kids had a bath since Saturday? It's time for supper again. Isn't it bedtime yet?

Can you see how my thoughts and circumstances felt like cliffs of insanity? I had thoughts like this rushing through my head all day. Sometimes it was like I was thinking in fast forward mode. One thought wouldn't end before the next round would begin. Sometimes they so thoroughly overlapped that I couldn't distinguish one from another.

It felt like my brain was just frying. When I was a kid the television programming would end for the day around midnight. The screen would display the American flag and the National Anthem would play. Then the screen would turn to a loud, obnoxious black-and-white snowy mess. That's what my brain and my life were like.

The incidents of my life were overwhelming and life altering. Christians who say we aren't supposed to let our circumstances affect us drive me nuts! Isn't that what God uses to teach and mold us? Don't we go through life learning to lean on God and not ourselves? How on earth could we do that if we lived aside from our circumstances? I've heard these things all my life: if we were just stronger, if we just trusted in the Lord, if we had more faith. What does that mean? I take God's word very seriously and literally. God says, "When you pass through the waters, I will be with you; and when you pass through the rivers, they will not sweep over you. When you walk through the fire, you will not be burned; the flames will not set you ablaze. For I am the Lord, your God, the Holy One of Israel…Since you are precious and honored in my sight, and because I love you, I will give men in exchange for you your life…Do not be afraid, for I am with you…" (Isaiah 43:2–5, NIV). If you haven't been through water or rivers or fire in your life, hang on! You will, and God will be there with you. We don't have to be strong. In 2 Corinthians 12:9 (NIV) Christ says, "My grace is sufficient for you, for my power is made perfect in weakness…" Proverbs 18:10 (NIV) says, "The name of the Lord is a strong tower; the righteous run to it and are safe." The Bible doesn't indicate that we get our strength from ourselves, but from God. In Colossians 1:29 (NIV) the apostle Paul writes, "To this end I labor, struggling with all his energy, which so powerfully works in me." Again, it's not us, it's him! Let's consider 2 Corinthians 4:16–17 (NIV), "Therefore we do not lose heart. Though outwardly we are wasting away, yet inwardly we are being renewed day by day. For our light and momentary troubles are achieving for us an eternal glory that far outweighs them all."

Instead of dwelling on our circumstances—for me they were my cliffs—I strongly believe that we need to thank God for helping us through them. Because of his help we are changed day by day, circumstance by circumstance. He gives us all his strength, patience, guidance, comfort, and love to see us through our circumstances. 2 Peter 1:3 (NIV) says, "His divine power has given us everything we need for life and godliness through our knowledge of him…" In essence, God's power gives us everything. He knows what we need way before we do. He knew I needed professional help, and through his power I got some. Often we don't realize what it is we need or want from God. Thankfully, he knows. When we pray, we are occasionally speechless. In our despair we just cry out and hope that God can make sense of our pain and anguish.

> "In the same way, the Spirit helps us in our weakness. We do not know what we ought to pray for, but the Spirit himself intercedes for us with groans that words cannot express. And he who searches our hearts knows the mind of the Spirit, because the Spirit intercedes for the saints in accordance with God's will." (Romans 8:26–27, NIV)

God even gives us things we don't want, but they are for our own good. Part of Isaiah 45:9b (NIV) reads, "Does the clay say to the potter, 'What are you making?'" Who are we to question God? He gave us life and salvation and a relationship with him. All we have to do is accept those gifts. Then we have to do what the old hymn says: "Trust and obey, for there's no other way to be happy in Jesus, but to trust and obey." That seems so easy. It almost makes trusting and obeying look pretty and neat. In our circumstances—good, bad and ugly—we are required to trust and obey. Job 2:10 (CEV) says, "…If we accept blessings from God, we must accept trouble as well…" My whole life, I truly thought I understood that concept. I honestly believed I would trust and obey and not question under any circumstances. My whole world was turned upside down at the hospital. Nothing has ever gotten my attention like my stint in the psych ward. I will be forever thankful that God was with me, and I knew it. I felt his presence like never before. Even in the craziest and scariest of places, I felt his compassion. I felt loved and protected in a brand new way.

Food for thought

"You're braver than you believe, stronger than you seem, and smarter than you think."

—Christopher Robin (from Winnie the Pooh)

The Fifth Floor

"The Lord *is my light and my salvation—whom shall I fear? The* Lord *is the stronghold of my life—of whom shall I be afraid? For in the day of trouble he will keep me safe in his dwelling; he will hide me in the shelter of his tabernacle and set me high upon a rock." (Psalm 27:1; 5,* NIV*)*

"Who shall separate us from the love of Christ? Shall trouble or hardship or persecution or famine or nakedness or danger or sword?" (Romans 8:35, NIV*)*

Before we left the emergency room, the needs–assessment woman took my husband to interview him. I was terrified of what they might ask him. I thought he might have known all along that I was sick and he would rat me out. I became so paranoid and scared that I could barely see straight. When he returned after just a short while, I was surprised that they didn't ask him much after all. Their main concern was the safety of our baby. They asked him if I seemed depressed. They also wanted to know his opinions on my relationship with the kids. They wanted to know if I'd bonded well with the baby or if I seemed to be a threat to him. I'm convinced they all thought I was lying to them. I never wanted to hurt the baby. I did have crazy thoughts and images about the baby, but they weren't my own. At the time, I wasn't sure I could clarify that well enough, so I just avoided the conversation. They also asked him a series of questions to decide if I was making all of it up. They learned it was not a hoax and that I was indeed sick. I couldn't fathom that someone would make up this story. What purpose would that serve anyone? Thankfully, my husband put their minds at ease. He reassured them I was quite sick, but not a danger to myself or the children.

It was nearly dinner time when the needs-assessment lady returned. She asked me if I felt comfortable going home. I did not, as I felt unable to care for the children. The thought of going home paralyzed me. I asked if I could stay and then signed papers to admit myself to the hospital. This was a turning point in my day.

When I signed the admittance papers, I assumed I was just giving them permission to take care of me. I had no idea that I was committing myself to the psychiatric unit of the hospital! My husband was of sound mind, and he didn't know either. No one ever explained to me what I was doing. I put on my hospital issued pajamas and followed a nurse. The ride up the elevator was silent. There was a huge BH across my green pajamas. I couldn't figure out, for the life of me, what the initials meant. A few hours later, I figured out that the BH stood for Behavioral Health. I was so exhausted that I still didn't fully comprehend what that signified. As the evening unfolded, I was furious to discover I'd been duped.

I knew I needed immediate help, but the psychiatric

unit didn't really seem to be the answer. I only experienced a few vague thoughts of suicide before entering the unit. They were almost like fantasies. I just wanted an escape from my incessant pain. I never really wanted to die. After spending a few hours in the hospital, death actually seemed appealing. In my psychotic fog, I wholeheartedly believed I would never leave the hospital. Once they escorted my husband and baby out of the ward, I thought my life as I knew it was over. As the door was locked behind them, I felt the intensity of my pain in every inch of my body. My life had become a disaster. I was convinced "they" were going to take my children into some sort of family services custody. I truly believed I wouldn't be able to see them again. To top things off, I wasn't sure they would want to see me again. I was scared to even guess what my husband was thinking or feeling. He just looked tired, exhausted from it all. My family leaving without me was a huge wake up call. I was on my own to fix this. God and I had some serious work to do.

After they left, I had to speak with yet another admitting nurse. She was special just to the psych unit. I had to answer at least one hundred questions. I just kept repeating the same thing all day long, just to different people. This lady's questions were a tad more serious and specific. She wanted to know if I had tried to kill anyone. She wanted to know if I had intentions of trying to kill anyone in the near future. Then came the final blow; I finally grasped the intensity of the situation. I was coerced into signing papers granting my permission to the staff to use restraints as needed. I had to give a contact name and number in case restraints were utilized. I thought that they knew something I didn't. I never read anything about women with PPD being restrained. Maybe my illness was going to unfold in a way that I couldn't foresee. I was sure, though, that I did want my husband contacted if they restrained me with some torture device. I fantasized about him busting in and rescuing me. It was a fresh experience for me, wanting to be rescued. I believed with all my heart that my husband would find a way.

After answering the millionth question of the day, I was escorted to my room. This was no ordinary hospital room. There was a bed and a table. There was no television. There were no posters or paintings or wallpaper. There was merely a bed with a pillow, sheet, and blanket; and a plain table and chair. There was one thing that really stuck out to me. There appeared to be a camera in the ceiling, pointed right at my bed. I had read about crazy people who became paranoid. I was convinced that was happening to me. I then checked out my bathroom. I was looking forward to taking a long, hot bath. There was no bathtub. There was a shower, toilet, and sink—all being watched by yet another camera. I surmised that other people in this place must have tried to kill themselves. They must have thought I wanted to kill myself. Unknowingly, I was put on suicide watch! I wanted to rewind the events of the day to try to clarify things. If I talked to the correct person, I knew they would transfer me. Unfortunately, they didn't.

The behavioral health unit of our hospital is located on the fifth floor. As far as I know, there isn't anything else on the floor. It appeared to be a mysterious place, where no one ventured to visit. It was as if we were in a vacuum, void of all outside contact. Time had a particular quality in that place; we were strangers to it. We were—literally—locked in to our physical and emotional surroundings. There was no escape. We had to deal with what was occurring or we couldn't go home. Even after months of freedom, I can call to mind the terror I felt physically and emotionally. The locked door presented fears I was unprepared to handle. I could no longer avoid my problems. To make matters worse, I could no longer avoid the people who were qualified to help me. I felt nauseous each time I saw an employee use a key to enter or exit the premises. Each time the door closed, the noise clamored in my head.

As I cried on my bed, a seemingly kind man came in to ask me more questions. He took me in the hallway to give me a tour of the place. There was a big white board on the wall. It displayed every patient's name, room number, social worker, nurse, and track. This nice man, Doug, tried to explain to me what all the classes were that I was required to take. There were two tracks: one for the low-functioning mentally ill patients, and one for people like me, who were just in crisis. Doug asked me if I knew what day it was and since I did, I was placed in the appropriate track. I concluded that people placed in the other track didn't know what day it was. For some reason, that heightened my fear. Doug explained that the two tracks of people would rarely intermingle. I was already terrified of therapy sessions. I had no clue what to expect. I was about to work my tail off in group sessions, with people I couldn't even look at.

Doug escorted me back to my room and asked me if I

had any questions. It was about time I got to ask a few! I told him I was seriously confused and didn't think I was in the right place. I pleaded with him to call my husband and let me go home. He said that was impossible. He further explained that I had to meet with a psychiatrist before I could ever be released. I had been waiting for more than twelve hours to meet with a psychiatrist. I felt frustrated and hopeless. Doug then went on to explain that I had to eat. He began talking to me like I was a little child. I became enraged. At that point, my anger wasn't helping my case. He just kept begging me to eat. He left to get me a snack. I went to the bathroom and starting vomiting. I don't recall ever crying so hard that I vomited. I just could not control myself. My stress level was through the roof, and I was stuck with this Doug nut. I realized someone was being paid to watch me in my bathroom as I vomited. Someone was probably drinking a soda, eating some chips, and watching a monitor in the office. I'm sure they were making notations in my chart. I was furious to think someone was watching me have a meltdown. It seemed so inhumane.

Doug came back with my snack, and I lost it. I really let him have it. I wanted to go home, and I wouldn't take no for an answer. There were significantly creepy people everywhere, and I was too timid to stay. He continued to talk to me like I was crazy. I wanted to throw the snack away, but I knew they would see me. At last, he left me alone with my snack in my plain room. Looking at the snack was at least something to do. It was much better than people watching at that place. I wasn't the least bit hungry. My stomach hurt intensely. I felt like someone had kicked it repeatedly, while wearing steel-toed shoes. I writhed in pain on my bed. A nurse came and gave me a sleeping pill so that I could rest and relax. The pill was almost an inch long. I wondered if the sleeping pill would put me in a coma. I wasn't so lucky.

Before going to sleep, I had one last task for the day. I had to use my breast pump in front of people. After giving birth, I didn't think anything could really embarrass me. Dozens of strangers had seen me mostly naked during the course of three hospital stays and three births. As a young twenty-something I had back surgery. During my recovery, my mother had to help bathe me for a week or more. That was terribly humbling. Once in my third trimester, I wore my maternity pants backwards to school. My remedial math kids tore me up over that one. I used to think these were embarrassing moments, but I was utterly debased as I checked my breast pump out of the office. I didn't understand why I couldn't keep my breast pump in my room. The nurse explained that the cords were a threat to my safety. As we walked down the hall back to my room, several pairs of eyes studied me and my black bag. I discerned that the strangers in the hall were the threat, not me. I was relieved to know that shortly my breast pump would be locked away. The humiliating part was having a nurse monitor me while I used my pump. She wasn't watching, per se, but she was there in the doorway, ever present. I was banned from closing my door. I had not even one ounce of privacy. The cameras were rolling as well. I was mortified that someone was watching me in the office via their television screen. I was scared that some of the characters in the hall might walk in at any moment. My situation became unbearable when I had to dump my milk in urine sample cups and carry them to the office to be refrigerated. The nurse at the window asked me to write the date on the cups. I paused momentarily, and she asked me if I knew what day it was. I didn't know how they expected me to remember the date under such duress. Thankfully, I recalled the date correctly and wasn't sent to the other side of the unit. I couldn't fathom what kind of scene was taking place over there. As I shuddered over what I had just endured, the sleeping pill did its job.

I slept for only a few hours before I woke up with a flashlight in my face. I nearly jumped out of my bed. I asked if something was wrong, and my good friend, Doug, whispered that he was just doing bed checks. From around ten P.M. to six A.M. someone would check my room every fifteen minutes. I'm still not convinced that was necessary. Nonetheless, it was procedure. As the night rolled on, I did fear for my safety. The guy across the hall was itching to do something really bad—I could feel it. I wondered if he'd ever killed anyone. He walked the halls, constantly trying to get away with disrobing. He made nasty comments and sang disgusting jingles he had concocted. He was the biggest guy in the place and wanted everyone to know it. He was totally off his rocker, and I doubted he knew what day it was. I refused to rest while this guy was being so obnoxious. Before the night was over, he set a fire in his room. I had small naps after the excitement, but didn't genuinely rest. Each time the light was shined in my face, my adrenaline started pumping again. I was reminded of where I was and who was lurking across the hall. The flashlights finally subsided and it was time to start the day.

I was exasperated when the nurse came to wake me up. She said I needed to eat and take a shower before the morning sessions began. I didn't eat, but I did shower. I just closed my eyes and forgot about the camera for a minute. It felt wonderful to have hot water wash over my swollen eyes and upset stomach. I longed to wash away the pain of the previous day. My body felt cleaner but my eyes and heart still hurt. A nurse from the lab came to draw my blood before I was fully dressed. She was super nice, and I thought she might be able to help me. I asked her if she would let me go home. Of course she didn't have the authority to release me, but I figured it didn't hurt to ask. After she left my room she quickly returned—hysterical. She was frantically looking for the tourniquet that she had just used. We went through my bed sheets and clothing. The tourniquet was nowhere to be found. I felt so bad for the nurse; she was just beside herself. As I finished dressing, I discovered the tourniquet under my bed. I ran to find the nurse so that I could reassure her that no one had gotten a hold of the ornery little piece of rubber. The relief in her eyes was immense.

Within minutes, I was escorted to my first therapy session. The program therapist explained a few things about what to expect at the meetings. Towards the end of the hall I located the exit, the locked door that symbolized my loss of freedom. My mind went into high gear as I thought of ways to escape through those doors. I was brought back to reality when the therapist showed me the electrocution room. I know that's not what it's called, but that's what I nicknamed it. She explained that electroshock therapy was quite successful in treating women with severe PPD. The look on my face must have said it all, because she tried to assure me that I wouldn't be visiting that room. It evoked feelings that were reminiscent of watching *The Wizard of Oz* as a small child. The all-powerful wizard hid behind the ominous curtain, terrifying little children. The electrocution room had the exact same aura to me. I was convinced that someone or something powerful and evil lurked behind that special door.

Our first therapy session of the day was strange. I was inundated with terms and procedures foreign to me. I was engulfed in the emotional gravity filling the room. All of the people at the meeting had been there before. Some of them seemed quite comfortable in that environment. I was so uncomfortable that I thought I might vomit. I struggled to avoid making eye contact. I dreaded bringing any attention to myself. I was about a minute late to the meeting, because I had to answer some questions for a nurse. The group was doing an icebreaker. We took turns reading goofy facts about coins, famous buildings, yarn, chewing gum, you name it. At the conclusion of our icebreaker, I felt more nervous than ever. I knew something challenging was ahead. We brainstormed misconceptions, labels, and negative stereotypes concerning mental health issues. I listened and found that I had developed many of these stereotypes in my own mind. I don't know where these ideas came from; perhaps they were inherited from my family or from our culture. We then learned of many famous people who were mentally ill, some from our generation and many from times past. We were supposed to feel normal because of other people's illness. I didn't feel the least bit normal or comforted by this information. Last on the agenda for this session, was something everyone else was quite used to. We had to draw a card out of a pile and answer a random question. I was rather intimidated as the pile came my way. My little card read, "Name one positive thing that happened yesterday." The floodgate opened wide with tears as I read the card aloud. I couldn't muster up an answer and all eyes were on me. I explained that yesterday was the day I arrived, and it had been like a never-ending nightmare since. After a few moments of silence, I thought of the one positive thing: I was there getting help. The idea of going through the process was causing me to panic internally and externally. I could no longer maintain any sense of composure. I fell completely apart in front of these strangers.

We had enough time to get a drink and then we came back for another group session. My tears would not stop, but my attitude had changed. I decided to utilize the professionals around me and do whatever it took to get out of there and home to my family. I was more determined in the following hours than I have ever been before. I was on a mission to do exactly what I was told: I would go to every meeting, meet with whatever unpleasant people I had to, eat whatever food they told me to, give milk, blood, and urine to anyone who asked for it. I busted out of my terrified shell and accepted the mission in front of me. I resolved during that session to just accept my fate and work with what I had. In the course of our session, we had to announce to the patients and the team of professionals what our goal was for the day. I wasn't really sure of where they were going with this, so I just listened and watched.

There was a guy named John who suffered from Bipolar Disorder and a few other unmentionables. He constantly talked about his imaginary friend Angel. He talked to her in the hall and in the therapy sessions. His goal for the day was to limit his discussions with her to once per session. One guy named Charles was cut up on his arms and neck. His cuts were quite fresh so I'm assuming he had recently attempted suicide. Just seeing him caused me to shudder. I could barely look at him. He was in such a fog of depression that he seemed to be living in an alternate dimension. His very presence gave me goose-bumps. I had never knowingly been around someone who had just tried to commit suicide. It made me so sad to see his body scarred and his face so downtrodden. His meager goal for the day was to take a shower. He didn't even come up with that on his own; the therapist suggested it. Somehow I grew to want to be around him. I felt like I didn't have it so bad. At least I wouldn't have scars on my body from this experience. There was a schizophrenic girl who absolutely shocked me. It was like watching a train wreck. I just couldn't quit staring at her. She had some other issues too, but I couldn't follow all of it. She had layers of diagnoses. Her goal for the day was to come up with a goal. She laid upside down in her chair and pulled her gum from her mouth in strings like a Kindergartner. She was a nervous wreck and verbally all over the place. I felt like I was running a 5K just being in the room with her. That meeting was mostly a blur for me. I had a difficult time listening because I wanted to conjure up an intelligent goal for the day. Since I was new to this, I wasn't really sure what to share. I didn't want people thinking I was stupid. I finally quit thinking and spoke from my broken heart. I expressed my goal with at least a dozen strangers that morning. My aim was to utilize all the help I could so that I could get well. I was going to keep crying and vomiting if that's what it took, but I was going to ask questions and dig in at the sessions. I wasn't going to sit back and let this take forever. I wanted to see my family no matter what it took. Fortunately, no one laughed at my goal. To make things even more comfortable, John had fallen asleep.

During the next group therapy session, I was relieved to know that I could be called out at any moment. I had been alerted that a nurse needed to see me to ask me some questions about my admittance papers. At this session, there was a new group leader. You could tell that this guy was an old pro. He was used to being emotionally beat up and verbally assaulted. John had forty ounces of Pepsi during the meeting, and he was raring to go. I had never seen someone act manic like this guy did. He truly flipped out on caffeine. I was surprised that they allowed him to have it in the first place. He was obnoxious and interrupted most of the meeting. Our leader eventually had to tell him to hush. Since I was in the hospital only days before Thanksgiving, we naturally talked about holidays. We made an extensive list of things that caused everyone stress at that time of year. We talked about the financial burdens of Christmas, sharing time between extended families, traveling with kids, expectations of parents, traditions that just couldn't be broken without a fight, remembering friends and family that had celebrated with us in the past, childhood memories of the holidays, etc. Then a pile of pictures was passed around the circle. We each had to draw out a picture from the pile and tell what that holiday meant to us personally. We were to discuss the good and bad memories associated with that holiday and any stress that particular time might bring. I drew Christmas and thought I might pass out from stress on the spot. The nurse came and called me out of the room. I was rescued right on cue!

To my disappointment, I was only out of the room for a minute, two at the most. For just that short time, I felt a little bit of freedom. I went back into the meeting room just as it was my turn. I talked about Christmas and how hard it was for me now. I spent so many years, literally waiting for my grandma to visit us at Christmas. It was the one time of year we went out for dinner. We either went to a steakhouse or a barbecue place. It was the biggest deal in the world to me as a little kid. Grandma did so many fun things with us. She would play cards, color, and paint; make cinnamon rolls and sugar cookies. I don't remember anything she ever taught me or said really; I just remember that she made me feel loved. Grandma's presence at Christmas was sacred in our family. When she

The Lifter of My Head

was too old to come, it just wasn't the same. I remember so many pictures of our family with Grandma at Christmas. Every year that Santa filled my stocking, I lovingly remembered that Grandma had made my special stocking. Even as a young child I remember treating my stocking with care. The first thing I reminisce about when it comes to Christmas is definitely Grandma.

Secondly, Christmas reminds me of pain. I am a person who always has high expectations of people, events, places, and life. I tend to get really excited and hopeful while others don't seem to. At one point in my life, I was a lot like Clark Griswold from *National Lampoon's Christmas Vacation*. In that movie, Chevy Chase plays a zealous dad who wants Christmas to be like a fairy tale. He pays careful attention to detail, not wanting to miss a thing. He puts nearly 50,000 lights on the house, wears all the holiday gear, has a beautiful turkey dinner, cuts down a pine tree so big it won't fit in the living room...you get the idea. Clark doesn't seem to let it bother him that he's the only one who is all fired up about Christmas. He wants to start great family traditions and he makes it his mission. I've had those same high hopes in the past, but it really hurts me deeply and personally when people aren't fired up like I am. I get excited about giving gifts, sending cards, making cookies and candies. As I age, I realize that Christmas is a much bigger deal to me than it is to most people around me. This sets me up for a perpetual letdown. Another thing I shared with the group was a painful memory from the previous Christmas. I had just found out that I was pregnant while we were visiting family. Typical of me, I was just bursting to share my news. It turned out to be one of the bigger mistakes of my life. I set myself up for failure. Not all of my family reacted positively to the news. Those negative reactions caused excruciating pain for months. Those were the memories of Christmas that I shared with my therapy group.

I then went on to talk about how special the birth of Jesus was to me. I talked about the first Christmas I had with my daughter and how I could understand a little more how Mary must have felt when she held Jesus for the first time. I could picture him as a baby and it was so precious to me. Some things in life can only be understood if you have a similar personal experience. Having a baby helped me see Jesus as a baby. He had to be fed, changed, and rocked. Mary didn't have the comforts of disposable diapers and wipes. I'm positive they didn't have La Leche League for support. I doubt she had a glider to sit in to rock the baby to sleep. It is amazing that he left the safety and comfort of Heaven to become a helpless babe in such primitive conditions. I cannot comprehend what a sacrifice that was for him. He cried and teethed. He might even have had ear infections and chicken pox. Having a child of my own made me see Jesus as a tangible human. Now each Christmas I can really celebrate the babe's arrival. I can really be thankful for Mary and Joseph's obedience to God and loyalty to each other. I am so glad that he came as a baby, not as an adult. Something about that makes his life even more believable and trustworthy. He is more real to me because of what Christmas acknowledges: his coming to earth as a human.

As we wrapped up our holiday meeting, I started to

feel a tremendous sense of guilt. It struck me like a bolt of lightning: I wasn't going to be able to go home to see extended family for the holidays. I would most likely still be in the psychiatric unit. I couldn't imagine they would release me. Even if I were allowed a pass for a few days, I could no longer hide my illness. At that point, it would be like trying to hide a broken leg. I felt incredibly guilty that I couldn't make the trip. Then God did a big thing! The doctor gave me orders to not travel during the holidays. God took care of me in a way that was brand new for me. He knew what I needed. I needed to stay home where I could begin to heal.

> In Psalm 27:1 and 5, (NIV) the Bible states, "The LORD is my light and my salvation—of whom shall I fear? The LORD is the stronghold of my life—of whom shall I be afraid? For in the day of trouble he will keep me safe in his dwelling; he will hide me in the shelter of his tabernacle and set me high upon a rock."

I was in the middle of my day of trouble. God kept me safe! He hid me in his shelter. I experienced his love and felt his protection envelop me in that craziest of places. I felt him setting me high upon a rock. I was aware of God's involvement in my circumstances and it gave me a fresh hope that I so desperately needed. I had to know this wasn't the end for me. I was on my way to recovery, and God let me know it. I was starting to feel his love and peace as only he can give. I knew without any doubts that he was with me. I was reassured as I recalled, "Who shall separate us from the love of Christ?" (Romans 8:35a, NIV).

I was sure that Christ was in the psychiatric unit with me. Even the most bizarre situation didn't scare Jesus away.

    The next group session proved to be the most interesting. It started out with this guy named Travis. He was in the hospital for a steroid-induced fit he threw. Apparently the drugs made him psychotic. He was probably about nineteen years old and thought he knew everything. I think most of us suffer from that misunderstanding in our teenage years. He proceeded to tell the majority of us in the room that we were just wallowing in our self-pity. All but two of the people were suffering from some form of depression. I decided to become our spokesperson. I couldn't let this kid tell us that we were choosing to be depressed. I said a really terrible thing as I lashed out in pain. I told Travis that he really was crazy if he thought I chose to be in the hospital. I really let him have it for a few minutes. All of my fellow "depressees" were proud of me for standing up to him. From the looks of things, Travis was a regular on the fifth floor. He was quite used to pushing people around and mouthing off whenever he felt like it. Most people were too scared or traumatized to even deal with him. I couldn't let him continue to verbalize his hurtful and ignorant opinions. He was convinced that everyone had to have a specific reason for their depression, and they simply were avoiding their true issues. One of our group leaders finally piped in after this comment. She attempted to explain to him that depression was significantly deeper than that. As I too learned, depression has many levels, varied root causes, and numerous solutions.

    The notion I got that day, was that no one could really

understand what I was personally undertaking. No one but God could truly understand. Sure, other women could relate because they had babies, some had even had postpartum depression; however, none of the other people on the fifth floor were currently suffering from PPD. Medical doctors, therapists, psychologists, psychiatrists, and even nurses do have a firm grasp of the illness. Unfortunately, PPD manifests itself differently in each case. There are a lot of symptoms that women share, but they sure do vary in frequency and intensity. I discovered during that session that I couldn't make Travis or anyone else understand what I was experiencing. Once I relinquished that unrealistic expectation, I made it my number one goal to fully understand it for myself. I asked lots of questions and talked for an hour about my experiences. It was therapeutic to finally spill my guts about everything. It was as if time stood still so I could get it all out. I think God gave me a few extra minutes of counseling because he knew I needed it. I talked the professionals into staying for a few minutes more so I could talk. I needed to know I would heal. I needed to hear a healthcare professional affirm my belief. They explained that I was doing a great job at the therapy sessions. They pleaded with me to be patient and let things happen at a natural pace. I felt as if they understood my illness and I could trust them. But did they understand me?

God understood what I was facing, because he made me. He was the one who designed my brain and my hormones. He created the life that triggered my depression. He knew the ins and outs of my pregnancy and its aftermath long before the baby was conceived. How could I not fully trust that he perceived my pain? Psalm 31:7 (NIV) says, "I will be glad and rejoice in your love, for you saw my affliction and knew the anguish of my soul." God sees us and our pain. I desperately cried out to him for understanding and comfort. He answered me immediately. I was almost shocked by how comforted I felt in that uncomfortable place. I sensed a deeper understanding of Psalm 91:4 (NIV), "He will cover you with his feathers, and under his wings you will find refuge; his faithfulness will be your shield and rampart." Who on earth, besides English majors, knows what a rampart is? Webster's New World Dictionary provides two definitions: 1) a fortification consisting of an embankment, often with a parapet built on top 2) a means of protection or defense; a bulwark. Those definitions forced me to look up more words! A parapet is a wall or bank used to screen troops from frontal enemy fire. Can't you just picture God screening fire for us? He screened fire from the wacky guy across the hall from me. He kept me safe from a very dangerous man. Even dearer to me is the picture of God as our bulwark. A bulwark provides defense or protection for someone or something. Until you have been terrified, you really can't grasp how precious that reassurance from God is. There was one man who remained in the ward for only about an hour. The police had to remove him. He was out of his mind on heroin. He had just tried to kill someone who was being treated in the emergency room downstairs. I had every intention of kicking out a window and jumping out if this guy wasn't sedated. I was alarmed and unnerved by this guy.

The Lifter of My Head

I knew I had to get away from him. Psalm 91:11–12 (NIV) says, "For he will command his angels concerning you to guard you in all your ways; they will lift you up in their hands, so that you will not strike your foot against a stone." God commanded his angels in major fashion. I quickly gave up my idea of jumping out the window. I prayed that God would protect me and get that man out of there. He did protect me. He protected everyone from the threats of that maniac. I felt supernatural protection for the first time in my life. As my preacher friend, Steve Miller, says, "If that don't light your fire, your wood's wet!" I was excited at the prospect of God doing what he said he would do. I believed him and trusted him fully.

The end of my stint in the psychiatric unit was all but uneventful. After thirty-five hours in the hospital, I met with the psychiatrist. She only asked me a handful of questions. Then, she told me I would be going home! She laughed as she skimmed my chart. Apparently, numerous people had noted in my chart that I wanted to go home. There was a strange lady that lurked the halls, taking notes of what we were doing every time she passed our room. I often told her that I wanted to go home. I'm sure she was annoyed with me. I might have even mentioned to the maintenance man that I wanted to go home. I was determined to go home before Thanksgiving. Since I seemed to be harmless, the doctor decided I could go home. She insisted that I needed lots of help, but I didn't have to stay locked in the hospital. I couldn't wait to get out of my room; I needed to call my family. After I called my husband, I prepared to go to my next session. A nurse came and explained my discharge papers to me. I was in utter shock. I assumed I was going home, but not that minute. I ran to the phone and my husband about fell over when I shared my news. He was just as ready as I was for this to all be over.

I skipped the next session as I prepared to go home. It was just recreational time anyway. It was during those precious minutes that God revealed himself in a huge way. A worker in the ward came and spoke with me. I was so elated to be leaving that I was unable to process much of what she said to me. Let me assure you, she was my angel, sent straight from God. She had been praying for me. She said she would continue to pray for me. She shared Scriptures and touching sentiments. I was flooded with intense gratitude. God provided a real person to speak with me, to pray for me, and to hug me. Even better, I had someone to say goodbye to. I had no desire to say anything to anyone else as I left. I wanted to stay under the radar at all costs. But for the purpose of closure, I needed to say goodbye to the person who I connected with the most. She assured me that I was ready to face the real world. She told me I was in good hands with the outpatient doctors I would be meeting. Her words of encouragement were more than I could have bargained for. I was ready to go home, but God knew what I needed. He knew I needed to have this conversation. I had to know someone understood me on a spiritual level. I had a renewed perspective concerning all that happened. I came to the conclusion that the whole world wasn't out to punish me. I also determined that God was big, bigger than I had given him credit for.

We had our routine afternoon meeting about rules,

concerns, and questions in the lounge. I sat still, trying not to grin or look at anyone. A huge fight was about to break out about who ate all the ice cream in the freezer. Just when it was starting to get heated, I saw my husband in my periphery. A nurse came and quietly called my name. I tiptoed out of the room, avoiding any eye contact. Since there was a fight, no one saw me leave. I was shaking as I reunited with my three children. As we walked down the hall, I saw the locked door. I was leery that someone might change their mind about me. I clung to my children as a nurse unlocked the door. I trembled as we rode on the elevator. When I took my first breath of fresh air, I thought I might collapse. I felt free, but uneasy. I had a renewed sense of hope for the future. I had successfully left the 5th floor with no intentions of ever returning.

Food for thought:

"If Jesus gives us a task or assigns us to a difficult season, every ounce of our experiences is meant for our instruction and completion if only we'll let him finish the work. I fear, however, that we are so attention-deficit that we settle for bearable when beauty is just around the corner."

—Beth Moore, Christian author and speaker

"Great hope makes great men."

—Thomas Fuller, English clergyman and historian

Post-Traumatic Stress

"For God has not given us a spirit of fear, but of power and of love and of a sound mind." (2 Timothy 1:7, NKJV)

The first moments outside of the psych unit were stressful. I was sick and scared, yet ecstatic to be released. I dreaded the path I was on; I knew healing was ahead, but I couldn't yet grasp it. Hard work and heartache were certain. Driving to our house was excruciating. I expressed to my husband that I didn't want to ever speak of the hospital. I was in utter shock at what I had experienced. I witnessed behaviors I had only read about in psychology textbooks. I was locked in a ward with psychotics and drug users. Suicidal and homicidal patients had surrounded me. Real, hurting people were abundant. I couldn't get their stories, scars, or faces out of my head.

The first thing I did when we got home was sit in a bubble bath. I tried to wash off the yucky feeling I had. The long, hot bath did nothing to soothe my nerves. I laid down on my bed and wept. It's all I could do. My husband just sat and listened for what seemed like hours. Not only was I miserably ill, I had just been exposed to some terrifying experiences and people. I hyperventilated emotionally and physically. I could not compose myself.

As the early days out of the hospital passed, I was contacted by someone from my insurance company. She set up appointments for me to meet with a psychiatrist and psychologist. In addition, I had a case worker who checked in on me, every other day, for a few weeks. I felt like I was in good hands for the time being. I had no expectations upon my first visit to the psychologist's office. But when I walked in, I freaked out. It was like I was back at the hospital. There were mentally ill people everywhere. Mental health professionals were coming out of the woodwork. When I signed in with the receptionist, I started sweating and crying. I could not look up at anyone. I started biting my fingernails and tapping my feet. I rocked back and forth, itching my arms and legs. Then I heard the deafening noise that stopped me dead in my tracks: the sound of a locked door. I panicked when I realized that patients and doctors were beyond the waiting room, behind locked doors. On the left, there was a locked door. On the right, there was a locked door. I felt like I had been duped once again. I was confident that whatever was going to happen was going to be bad.

I met my psychologist and was instantly paralyzed. I am a fairly confident person when I speak to others. I was feeling like a mouse trying to connect with an elephant. As the initial visit got underway, I realized that this woman had the power to put me back on the 5th floor. She had a power over me that was stifling. I struggled to share with her. I never lied, but I withheld information at times. I was thankful that she was so brilliant. She knew when I was filtering information or withholding anything important. Each week that I met with her, I became less and less afraid.

It took several months for me to trust my psychologist fully. I didn't believe I had a choice. The process itself was foreign to me. I figured I'd lie on a couch and she'd ask me questions about my mother. I sat on a chair, and we didn't talk about my mother at all! Seriously, I was terrified of the power she had in my life. I couldn't even concentrate on getting well through therapy. I imagined that she would one day send me back to the psychiatric unit. Once she realized my hang-up, she reassured me I wasn't going back. That is when therapy started to change my life. It changed my perspective on my present illness, my past troubles, and my future hope. She knew who I was on a significantly deep level. It was funny how well this stranger knew the intricate workings of my mind. Her ability to read me set me at ease somehow. I felt God directly comforting and teaching me through her. My negative thinking patterns were slowly transformed to positive ones. I anticipated healing; it came in spurts.

For a while, therapy seemed to be the cure-all. As long as I had someone to hear me, I felt confident that I would be okay. It was when I started taking steps backward, that I saw the complexity of my illness. I would have good weeks and bad weeks. Then the bad weeks started out numbering the good ones. I was doing the work required of me, so it made no sense that I was backpedaling. It irritated and angered me to have come so far only to go back so far. That's how it is with postpartum depression. It took a long time for my medication to fully work. My mind needed a long time to heal. I harbored a tremendous amount of anger. I wanted to be completely well in a matter of weeks. It just didn't happen. I would take a few steps forward and many steps backward. I would get myself together, just in time to fall apart again. Eventually, though, I saw that the process was working.

One huge issue I had to work out was the post-traumatic stress I was unsuccessfully coping with. My therapist and I didn't spend much time on this issue. Unfortunately, I suffered with this for several weeks. I was never diagnosed with Post-Traumatic Stress Disorder, but I did have stress related to trauma. According to the National Institute of Mental Health, "Post-Traumatic Stress Disorder (PTSD) is an anxiety disorder that can develop after exposure to a terrifying event or ordeal in which grave physical harm occurred or was threatened…Many people with PTSD repeatedly re-experience the ordeal in the form of flashback episodes, memories, nightmares, or frightening thoughts, especially when they are exposed to events or objects reminiscent of the trauma…PTSD is diagnosed when symptoms last more than one month…" I constantly relived the trauma of the hospital and the events that led up to it. I didn't dream about the events, which shocked me. But many things triggered a stress response for me. I relived the morning I went to the emergency room every time I got in the bath tub. Sometimes just being in the bathroom bothered me. I wondered if someone was watching me. Every time I heard the door shut at the doctor's office, I felt physically sick. Sometimes, locks on doors at my own house bothered me. Seeing pregnant women or baby clothes would make me break down. When women shared their labor and delivery stories my blood pressure would skyrocket. I couldn't appropriately deal with anything related to pregnancy, childbirth, or healthcare facilities. It took almost a year for those fears and anxieties to wane.

Most of that part of my illness is a blur to me now. I don't recall how I got through it every day. I do know that my focus was on thankfulness. I began to thank God I wasn't locked up. I also thanked him for my locked doors! (Many days I wondered if some of my hospital buddies would find my house.) I gave him praise for saving my life. I thanked him that I could take a relaxing bubble bath and that no harm would come to me, no crazy thoughts would enter my mind. Even though I couldn't always be fearless in my bathroom, the episodes of anxiety were becoming less frequent. I saw progress. Each time I saw my friend who miscarried, I thanked God, in advance, for her next pregnancy and baby. I asked God to heal my traumatic delusions of miscarriage. It took a very long time for me to come to terms with my fears concerning my imagination. My mind went through some terrifying events. I never denied my fears, I just re-thought them. I focused on being thankful instead of fearful. I had to ask God to give me this mind-set. I know it was from him, because my natural reaction was fear. I clung to the verse, 2 Timothy 1:7 (NKJV), "For God has not given us a spirit of fear, but of power and of love and of a sound mind." I was confident that through God's help, I could quit being scared, and start feeling his power. Over time, my post-traumatic stress vanished. I slowly regained the sound mind that God gave me.

Food for thought:

"The greatest weapon against stress is our ability to choose one thought over another."

—William James,
American philosopher and psychologist

The Unquiet Mind

"Don't fret or worry. Instead of worrying, pray. Let petitions and praises shape your worries into prayers, letting God know your concerns. Before you know it, a sense of God's wholeness, everything coming together for good, will come and settle you down…" (Philippians 4:6–7, Msg)

"The LORD your God is with you, he is mighty to save. He will take great delight in you. He will quiet you with his love, he will rejoice over you with singing."(Zephaniah 3:17, NIV)

During my senior year of high school, I took my first psychology class, Abnormal Psychology. I was drawn to it like a moth to a flame. It fascinated me to learn about the mind. My friends and I would diagnose different kids and teachers in our school. One of our track coaches screamed of Bipolar Disorder, our art teacher was obsessive–compulsive; our volleyball coach had an oedipal thing. I wanted to get my hands on the infamous DSM-IV so I could continue my diagnosing with more authority. The DSM-IV is the diagnostic criteria for the most common mental disorders published by the American Psychiatric Association and used by mental health professionals in the United States. I was convinced a paranoid schizophrenic sat behind me in Trigonometry class. Our little club of Future Psychologists of America only had the intention of entertaining ourselves, we meant no harm. Little did I know that one day I would struggle to identify my own mental illness.

My depression had so many layers of symptoms. At

times I couldn't separate my depression from my anxiety and it stressed my brain to even try. I came to terms with the fact that I wasn't a psychologist and tried to let my real psychologist do the work. I falsely believed that I required intellectual insight into my illness. I read every article, blog, and book I could get my hands on that covered any of my symptoms. "You aren't alone" is a common theme I discovered. It didn't bring me any comfort to read of famous people with mental illness. These famous or influential people have struggled with all types of mental illnesses: Charles Dickens, Abraham Lincoln, Winston Churchill, Ludwig van Beethoven, Vincent Van Gogh, Sylvia Plath, Edgar Allen Poe, Kurt Cobain, Robin Williams, and Jim Carrey. I found minimal solace in knowing that others suffered as I did. A few of these folks committed suicide. That wasn't so encouraging. No matter what I read, I still maintained that I had somehow detected a new strain of depression. I continued to believe I was alone.

    I wanted to know definitive answers to all the basic questions: who? what? when? where? why? and how? Who suffers from PPD? There's a misconception that it's usually in first time moms because they have certain ignorance about motherhood. What a nonsensical thought. Postpartum depression hits whomever it will. Being unprepared for motherhood can make it difficult. Depression is way more than difficult. It's an illness, not a rough week. I've literally had people tell me, "Well I was nervous too, when I first went home from the hospital. I cried when my husband went back to work. I was so tired that first month." Good for you! Most of us have been *there*, but that is not depression.

What causes PPD? Hormones are a cop out, aren't they? What chemicals in my body have me so messed up? When did this happen? Did it start while I was in labor? When was the launch sequence activated? Could I have stopped it? Where was the help I needed? Where were the real answers to be found? Why me, Lord? If you've never said that before, your time might be coming! (I never thought I'd say it either.) I begged God to reveal to me why I needed to go through this insane time. And finally, how did this happen? Did I eat too many cheeseburgers and shakes? Was it because I didn't take my prenatal vitamins regularly? There had to be answers. So I read and read until my head ached. Finally something clicked.

In our Abnormal Psychology class we were introduced to the concept of fight or flight. Our body has a primitive system in place by which we respond to threats to our safety. When the acute stress response is activated, we tend to perceive everything in our environment as a threat. When we are faced with an attack on our well-being, we do one of two things instinctively: we face the threat— "fight," or we avoid it— "flight." It is natural and normal for us to react in this manner. What is not normal is to feel afraid and upset most of the time without any threat. Many illnesses and situations lead people to have an overactive fight or flight response. In my case, it played a monumental role in my PPD.

My fight or flight instinct would turn into a panic attack in a matter of seconds. In my therapy sessions, I learned that I could be facing a trigger for my panic attacks and immediately jump to a catastrophic thought. At first

I thought that sounded so dramatic but it really explained what was happening with my thought process. I really toiled to accurately identify and describe my tormenting thoughts. Here are a handful of facts and symptoms associated with the most common catastrophic thoughts and reasons not to fear them.[1]

1. Heart palpitations, increased pulse rate
   Catastrophic thoughts: What if my heart stops? It cannot take this stress. I might have a heart attack. Truth: The heart is composed of very strong muscles which can take much more than you believe. During a panic attack the heart can beat irregularly, and you can experience chest pain. An electrocardiogram taken during a panic attack is normal, although it shows that the heart beats more rapidly.

2. Dizziness, unsteady feeling
   Catastrophic thoughts: I will faint. What if I fall? Truth: Very few patients with panic disorder will faint. Your dizziness depends on, among other things, on a slight reduction of the blood circulation in the brain, and due to high muscle tension in the head and neck. This can also lead to an unsteady feeling. The heart will beat more rapidly, which increases the blood circulation and counteract any tendencies to faint.

3. Breathing difficulties, choking sensations
   Catastrophic thoughts: What if I stop breathing? I am choking. I can't breathe.

Truth: The chest muscles can tighten, which makes it feel heavier to breathe. There is no possibility of you tightening them until you choke. The brain has a reflex which controls the oxygen intake, and it will force you to breathe even if you try not to. In the rare case that you should faint, you will start breathing automatically. Breathing difficulties can also be a result of hyperventilation. This results in expiration of too much carbon dioxide. You can counteract it by slow abdominal breathing or, in acute cases, by breathing in a paper bag.

4. Feelings of unreality and de-realization
   Catastrophic thoughts: What if I lose control? I am losing my mind. The world around me seems funny.
   Truth: The lowered blood circulation in the brain results in some odd symptoms, such as disorientation and feelings of unreality. It does not mean that you are losing your mind. You will not hear voices or be subject to hallucinations during a panic attack, unless you have taken drugs. Most disorders with a disturbed behavior, such as psychosis or schizophrenia, develop gradually during a long period of time, and the person does not realize that something is wrong.

Automatic thoughts are ones that come and go at will. Most people are not aware of the influence these thoughts have on our well-being and our lives. A common objection against the importance of negative thoughts is that the anxiety should disappear once you have realized the connection. That is not the case, because these thoughts are automatic and affect feelings and bodily sensations which are not directly controlled by willpower. Both practice and power is required, first to detect the thoughts, then to re-evaluate them. For example, does a tennis player's game improve just because the coach tells him he hits the ball into the net too often?[2] It's highly unlikely that observation would change a thing. In the same way, it is not possible just to replace negative thoughts with positive ones, when you are anxious or depressed. That would be like trying to lie to yourself. You can try to replace the negative thoughts with questioning and realistic observations. To be successful though, you must identify the negative thoughts again and again and re-evaluate their accuracy. Catastrophic thoughts typically go hand in hand with panic disorder. So much centers around death e.g. in a heart attack, or losing control, or becoming insane. But with the passage of time and awareness of your thoughts, these things will pass. Not for one minute did I believe those awful things would pass for me. I counted on God to help me adjust to my new lifestyle. But I never imagined that my thought life could be so altered and healed.

Panic attacks and racing thoughts were terrifying phenomena to me. Immediately after leaving the hospital, I started experiencing panic attacks. Within a few more days, the racing thoughts flooded my mind. Mixing the two problems together made for a psychological and emotional nightmare. The panic attacks came one right after another for the first few days. With the passing of time, they slowed to fewer than ten a day. There were two significant triggers that activated my panic response: driving and reading. Driving was especially distressing. I would practically lose my mind while I was concentrating on where I was going, how I was to get there, and when was I supposed to arrive. I would suffer every time I got in the car. Another big trigger was reading. Any written word just stumped my brain. Trying to read anything was agonizing. I would sweat, pant, and get shaky as I tried to read simple things like my checkbook register or notes from my daughter's school. Reading e-mails and books, for example, was nearly impossible. I was unable to focus on the words. They ran together in a massive blur. Basic writing was incomprehensible. My eyes couldn't make sense of anything. The confusion would cause my heart to race. I felt muscle tension, chest pressure, stomach pains, and nausea. The symptoms of my panic attacks were overwhelming.

Ironically, as the severity of my attacks waned, I became proficient in how to cope with the symptoms. I learned to breathe deeper and slower. I grasped, through my talk therapy sessions, that I was in fact making my attacks worse by trying to stop them. I would get so upset by my oncoming attacks that I could actually heighten the symptoms. Often times, I would just be agitated or confused and that would make it worse. I would become aware of my upcoming attack. Just being aware of my symptoms could make my panic attacks just explode. Once I came to terms with my panic attacks, I could calmly ride them out as my therapist suggested. It helped to count and breathe; oftentimes closing my eyes made these routines even more effective. As I embraced this new problem, it slowly went away on its own.

I chose to quit worrying about my panic attacks and how deeply weird they were. I made a conscious decision to give the whole problem to God. I shared with him that I was scared and felt out of control. Somehow he quietly reminded me that he was in control all along, even when I wasn't. Miraculously I felt a new peace even in the midst of the worst of my attacks. I knew God was with me and would never leave me. I pictured him saddened by my pain instead of judging me. At first, I considered my anxiety to be a character flaw. When I fully grasped the medical nature of my condition, I let go of that silly idea. I chose to not feel self conscious around others. Does that mean I never was? No way! But with God's help, I soon felt more at ease and still in my spirit. My brain was calming down and so were my nerves. I felt as if God were settling my spirit, quieting me with his presence.

As soon as I got my panic attacks under control, another huge problem hit me like a Mack truck. I experienced racing thoughts day and night. According to Marcia Purse, from an online newsletter about Bipolar Disorder, racing thoughts are quite complex.[3] She said, "Before I knew anything about Bipolar Disorder—much less than I myself had it—I called this sensation 'racy brain.' Thoughts and music would be zooming through my head so fast that sometimes I wanted to scream. If it was going on at bedtime, it could take me an hour or more of concentrating on word games to get myself to sleep. Racing thoughts are not just 'thinking fast.' They are thoughts that just won't be quiet; they can be in the background of other thoughts or take over your consciousness; they can gallop around in the sufferer's head like a carousel gone out of control."

Components of racing thoughts can include music, snatches of conversation from movies or television or books, one's own voice or other voices repeating a phrase or sentences again and again, or even rhythms of pressure without any "sound" in the thought. The phenomenon called racing thoughts is distinctly different from "hearing voices," which is a symptom of schizophrenia, schizoaffective disorder, severe mania, or other psychotic disorders. Racing thoughts can be a symptom of mania, hypomania or a mixed episode, but unlike some other symptoms of these moods, can also occur during depression or an anxiety disorder. Sometimes racing thoughts are accompanied by a pounding heart or pounding pulses, including drumming in the ears. Some people are gifted at multi-tasking; I'm not one of those people. I can only do one thing well at a time. If I try to multi-task, I end up with absolutely nothing accomplished. That exact same thing occurred with my thought life. For example, I would be trying to write the bills. Looking at the numbers and words would spark me thinking about other paperwork that needed to be done. Then I would start seeing all the print on the desk. It all ran together like one big blur. While being unfocused on print was disturbing, so was my inability to comprehend the spoken words around me. The kids seemed to be in my head screaming gibberish. The television and radio were just as unnerving. I couldn't differentiate between what was background noise and what was important. It was as if I were wearing a hearing aid that was turned all the way up, humming for the whole world to hear. The fan on the refrigerator was deafening at times, whereas I couldn't even make out what my son was asking for in the kitchen. I just couldn't focus on any one thing or tune out unimportant noises. It was frustrating to not be able to reduce the number of thoughts I had rushing through my head. It was maddening to not be able to quiet them.

In some ways my frantic mind mimicked a few symptoms that accompany Bipolar Disorder. I didn't experience the highs typical of Bipolar Disorder, but I did express some of the mania and depression. Life seemed so intense. My environment appeared so much brighter and so much darker at the same time. I experienced everything in the world so much more intensely than everyone else. I would often express my discomfort, looking for confirmation from my family members. I was always hotter than everyone else. Noises bothered me that no one else even noticed. Lights and sounds tortured me. I couldn't explain how annoying every single thing was. Everything was affected by my bizarre thoughts. I experienced an unspeakable pain, loneliness, and terror. It was like I was living in a different reality. My madness was now more real to me, almost tangible. The rushing thoughts kept overlapping. The fast ideas kept coming faster, creating an overwhelming confusion. The confusion led to irritability, anger, and more darkness. I felt completely alone in my madness.

In the midst of my mental chaos, my memory worsened, my sense of humor disappeared; but God never left me. I knew I couldn't will my mind to heal. I insisted that God would see me through this, and I just had to trust him. Jeremiah 17:7–8 (NIV) contains some powerful words, "But blessed is the man who trusts in the Lord, whose confidence is in him. He will be like a tree planted by the water that sends out its roots by the stream. It does not fear when heat comes; its leaves are always green. It has no worries in a year of drought and never fails to bear fruit." I clung to the knowledge that God was my confidence, my water during the drought, and he produced fruit in me even while I was sick! Psalm 55:22 (NIV) says, "Cast your cares on the LORD and he will sustain you; he will never let the righteous fall." It is easy to skim over those words and not really notice their significance. According to Webster's Dictionary, sustain means the following: "1. to keep in existence; keep up; maintain or prolong; 2. to provide for the support of; specifically to provide sustenance or nourishment for; 3. to support from or as from below; carry the weight or burden of; and 4. to strengthen the spirits, courage, etc. of; comfort; buoy up, encourage." For the first time, I cherished the thought that God would sustain me. In the middle of PPD you just cannot see any end to the pain. You really don't feel that you will recover. Fortunately, I had God sustaining me each and every day. God kept me in existence; he maintained my life while I couldn't do a thing for myself. He took care of my kids while I had to concentrate on getting well. He supported our family and carried the burden of my illness. I firmly believe that he sheltered my children from the pain of my problems. Despite what some professionals have argued, I don't think they suffered as a result of my depression. I believe God guarded them as he endured this season of my life with me. He came alongside my husband and gave him tremendous strength, courage, and energy. While we were in survival mode for months, my husband seemed at peace. Only God can give that kind of peace, a sort of stillness in the storm.

My mind remained unquiet for a few more months and my faith was strenuously tested. I pleaded with God to just declare, "Time's up! It's all over now." In retrospect, it was to my benefit that God made me trust him in an all-consuming way. There were numerous people in my life that had to deal with my illness. When something like this happens to you, it really sorts out your relationships. Intense circumstances tend to separate the men from the mice. I was shocked at the family and friends who really supported me during that time. I was devastated by those who didn't. The love and help that I received far outweighed any apathy that surrounded me. The good was so overwhelming that I didn't have time to notice the bad. I prayed daily that God would bring people into my life to meet every single need I had. God never failed me. I cried out to him for help and he always sent it. God never directly knocked on my door, called me, e-mailed me, or brought me food. He did, however, send people to me. I will forever be grateful for my friends who responded to the needs of our family. I know that God intervened and prompted some hearts. According to author Max Lucado,

"The people who make a difference are not the ones with the credentials, but the ones with the concern."[4] Simple, unashamed, unwavering obedience to God yields such huge results. God can use anyone as long as they are willing. Most people never knew the intensity of my illness, nor did they need to, but they obeyed God and helped our family in time of crisis. I believe God will richly reward them for "it is more blessed to give than receive," according to Acts 20:35b (NIV).

An unquiet mind is a sad mind. I didn't feel like I was participating in the real world. As my symptoms intensified, I really detached from the world around me. I don't know if too many people comprehended my withdrawal, I'm sure I hid it well. For a few short months, I lived in the bubble of my sick mind. I did live in fear, but not permanently. I knew God would see me through it all, but I was scared. If a mentally ill person tells you they aren't scared, I question their integrity. I knew God was in charge of it all, but fear of the unknown kept creeping back into my mind. Thanks be to God; he didn't leave me alone. He didn't leave my mind to further decay either. His presence never left me and as a result, I found peace and healing during the toughest times of my postpartum months.

Food for thought:

"Some of the hurts you have cured, and the sharpest you still have survived, But what torments of grief you endured, from evils which never arrived!"

—Ralph Waldo Emerson, American author and poet

Friends God Gave Me

"A friend loves at all times, and a brother is born for adversity." (Proverbs 17:17, NIV)

"...serve one another in love." (Galatians 5:13b, NIV)

"Bear one another's burdens, and so fulfill the law of Christ." (Galatians 6:2, NKJV)

"Therefore, as we have opportunity, let us do good to all people, especially to those who belong to the family of believers." (Galatians 6:10, NIV)

God created us to be in fellowship with one another. We were never meant to be alone. We were meant to serve, rejoice, cry, and grow with one another. It's spelled out clearly in the Scriptures. But do we do it? Do we really understand it? Specifically, what does service look like? To keep things simple, I looked up the word service in my daughter's *Scholastic Children's Dictionary*. Service is simply work that helps others. While I had the book open, I searched for the definition of helpful; it just means willing to help. For most of us working to help others is easy enough to understand. It's the willingness that can be tough. It makes us acknowledge where our focus is. Is it all about me or is it about others? Matthew 25:35–40 reminds me that whatever we do for other people it is as if we were doing it for Christ himself. That's huge! By loving others, we are loving Christ.

We search for these huge acts of service that we want to be a part of, all the while missing many opportunities. Rick Warren writes in *The Purpose Driven Life*, "Great opportunities often disguise themselves in small tasks." I can relate to the feeling of wanting to do something big. I recall attending a Newsong concert with a dear teacher friend of mine in Tyler, Texas. It was the first time I was exposed to information about World Vision. I was so on fire for God and for feeding poor kids that I could hardly contain myself. I wanted to take over World Vision and go on tour with Newsong until every Third World kid was fed! How silly was that?

Our interim pastor spoke once on this overzealousness. Many of us have big causes we see ourselves fitting in with. These might very well be worthy aspirations. It's quite easy to get excited about big things. It's not as appealing to do work that no one sees but God. Lots of people are lining up to be seen, but few choose to do the behind-the-scenes work. Sure, Jesus did big things; he is still in the business of doing big things. But Jesus did a load of small things. He washed feet, played with little children, cooked breakfast on the shore, visited with prostitutes and dishonest people. Jesus said to be holy because he is. I am sure he wants us spending more time in our sphere of influence than he does in our sphere of concern. In Stephen Covey's national bestseller, *The 7 Habits of Highly Effective People*, he explains this phenomenon as the circle of influence vs. the circle of concern. He spells out that the first good habit is proactivity:

"Another excellent way to become more self-aware regarding our own degree of proactivity is to look at where we focus our time and energy. We each have a wide range of concerns—our health, our children, problems at work, the national debt, nuclear war. We could separate those from things in which we have no particular mental or emotional involvement by creating a Circle of Concern. As we look at those things within our Circle of Concern, it becomes apparent that there are some things over which we have no real control and others that we can do something about. We could identify those concerns in the latter group by circumscribing them within the smaller Circle of Influence. Proactive people focus their efforts in the Circle of Influence. Reactive people, on the other hand, focus their efforts in the Circle of Concern."[1]

These two circles might coincide, but the bottom line is this: we all have people in our lives—neighbors, co-workers, children, spouses, family members, clerks at the store, acquaintances, the parents of our children's friends; you name it, we've got them. We have people we come in contact with all the time. That's who Christ called us to serve. He might call us to something else, something "big." But for now I want to focus on what I know I have to do. I want to be obedient in my life as I know it. If I could just be obedient in my daily life, that would be big! As Beth Moore says about the prayer of Jabez from 1 Chronicles, "Why do we want God to expand our territories when we aren't being faithful in our own backyard?"[2] As a woman, you know a woman you can serve. You most likely know someone who has a child. You probably know a woman who can't have a child. You know women who have tons of kids and need loads of help! You might know someone suffering with PPD. Surely, you know a single woman. You probably know a younger woman who could use some guidance. I am positive you know a woman who could use prayer. No matter who you are, you know someone. Serve that person as if you were serving Christ. As a child of the eighties, I'll never forget Nike's best slogan to date: "Just do it."

One of the keys to fellowship is walking side by side with people as they experience life. Romans 12:15 (NIV) says, "Rejoice with those who rejoice; mourn with those who mourn." Hebrews 3:13a (NIV) says, "But encourage one another daily..." Romans 15:5, (NIV) states, "May the God who gives endurance and encouragement give you a spirit of unity among yourselves as you follow Christ Jesus..." Acts 2:45–47 (NIV) describes the fellowship of the early church,

> "Selling their possessions and goods, they gave to anyone as he had need. Every day they continued to meet together in the temple courts. They broke bread in their homes and ate together with glad and sincere hearts, praising God and enjoying the favor of all the people. And the Lord added to their number daily those who were being saved."

God expects us to be in fellowship with one another. We long for authentic friends who will unconditionally love us yet hold us accountable. God would love for us to have deeper friendships along our life's journey.

My life has been at times full of friends, and at times

void of friends. The one friend who has been constant is Jesus. He has been my never-changing, never-leaving companion. In the years prior to our most recent move to Minneapolis, I was often friendless. For a couple of years I was in a vacuum with my husband and kids, void of much outside contact or love. Sure, we went to church. But we were empty and sad, mostly taking up space in a pew. People didn't appear to care much if we were there or not. We attended a church that was on its death bed. Oh sure, the usual crowd showed up week after week. Unfortunately, they didn't have the first clue as to how they were supposed to act as God's people.

One of my father figures, George Roach, lives in the middle of nowhere in Missouri. I happen to miss the middle of nowhere from time to time! Anyway, he coordinated missions, working with all the local churches to perpetuate fellowship and mission work. But what impressed me was his ability to speak to my heart. He spoke simply so I could understand but he was never simplistic. I started to write a book titled *The Churches We Need and Why We Don't Have Them*. I really wanted to unearth the reasons why our local churches were really missing the mark. One Sunday, George was preaching and he gave me the answer I'd been pursuing. Churches can thrive if they have two things: a passion for Christ and a genuine compassion for people. Let that soak in for a minute. How profound. From that moment on I knew it was my responsibility to quit waiting on all the lazy Christians. It was my turn. I dove in, working my tail off in that church and community. Nothing much changed in that place, but I did. God worked a miracle in my heart. We left that community with a few last-minute friends who will always be in our hearts and God-willing, our lives. I look back on that time as a huge learning experience. I am so grateful that I was friendless for a couple of years. I saw God as my friend for the first time ever. I read my Bible as if I was hearing straight from God. Previously, the Bible felt like stories about other people or words of wisdom I'd never grasp. The Scriptures were alive to me, and so was my relationship with Jesus. It would be a few years before I realized how precious a learning experience this was.

I attended a Hearts at Home conference in Rochester, Minnesota, after moving to the Twin Cities. In one of the breakout sessions, the speaker Allie Pleiter, described different kinds of friends that God plants in the garden of our lives. (I'll let you know up front that I don't know the first thing about gardening, so her comparing different types of friends to various flowers was lost on me. I'm sure some of you would greatly benefit from her beautiful floral parallels!) I wrote down every word Allie said, not knowing when I might need to return to these nuggets of truth. I love taking notes. Not much else in the world makes me quite as happy. (We never did get to that in my therapy sessions!) As I took my notes about friends, I found myself thinking about different friendships that had come and gone, mostly ones that had gone.

I have had several groups of friends who have come and gone. I have a very precious picture by my front door that reminds me of some wonderful times with dear friends in Kansas City. It reads, "Some people come into our lives and quickly go. Some stay for awhile and leave footprints on our hearts and we are never the same." The women who signed the back of that picture will never comprehend how special that has been for me over the years. I recall the laughter and tears and prayers. I still recall my dear friend from that group telling me she was pregnant with her first child. I had never had a friend who was pregnant before. I was so thrilled I didn't even know what to do. I remember watching her newborn son in the hospital. I cried with happiness for their family. I often look at that plaque and notice it needs dusting. But some days it brings tears of joy to my eyes. I am so blessed to have such a rich history with these friends. Unfortunately, I have lost touch with most of those women. We've all scattered to different churches, some of us even different to states. But God truly blessed me with those women and their influence. I had never earnestly clung to my friends until I went through my crisis months. I remembered what Allie had said and dug out my notes to review. It's amazing that I could look at all of my friendships and relate to what she had said years ago. She elaborated on several kinds of friends: the twin, the sparkler, the rock, the "been there" friend, the challenging friend, and the best-ever friend.

Allie described the "twin friend," someone with whom you have a mutual experience. She used Sam and Frodo from *The Lord of the Rings* as an example. These types of friends give us a sense or normalcy, that what we are going through is okay. The only downside of this type of friend is that they can't give us any objective perspective, since we're in the same boat. For me, my twin friends are numerous. I am blessed to have lots of women currently in my life that are raising small children and still having babies. These aren't necessarily our closest friends, but they sure know what we're going through. God truly blessed me with twin friends when I had my baby. I assumed that since he was my third child no one would really get too excited about his arrival. I was completely wrong! I was flooded with e-mails, visits, food, phone calls, gifts, and support. My twin friends showed up *en masse*.

I learned so much from my friends when I had my third baby. I learned from their behavior how to truly love people. I know that some people are shy and have a hard time reaching out to others. We can't do everything for everybody, but we can do something for someone! All the things that we might think are insignificant can really add up and help others. I have numerous examples of things my friends did for me that I just have to share. Sometimes we aren't sure how to help so here are a few things I'll not soon forget. One friend from church called and asked me what I needed from the grocery store. Never in my wildest dreams had I imagined someone doing something so kind for me. I was so overwhelmed and tired, I couldn't fathom making a trip to the grocery store. I told her we could use some milk and she gently chastised me, reassuring me that she would get more items than that. When she realized I was so sleep deprived that I couldn't think straight, she started making suggestions. By the end of our conversation we had a list consisting of eggs, bread, cheese, fruit, orange juice, you name it and she had already thought of it. Getting those groceries on that exhausting day was a precious gift. That, my friends, is an example of how God met my needs that I hadn't even identified! Another friend came over one day and held the new baby. She told me to lie down while my preschooler napped, and she would entertain the baby. I didn't argue for one second! Did I sleep? No way. I was a complete insomniac at the time, but boy it felt good just to lay down. Sometimes my head felt like it weighed one hundred pounds in those early postpartum weeks. I was so tired I walked into walls and tripped over my own feet. What a priceless gift that friend gave! This same friend brought us a meal to eat, but even better, she brought snacks for the big kids. She brought a ton of grapes and homemade chocolate chip cookies. I was thrilled to have their favorite treats on hand. Lots of friends from church and the neighborhood brought us food. Lasagna was a staple in our house for about two weeks! Our family loves the animated movie *Madagascar*. One of the memorable lines from the movie is, "Don't bite the hand that feeds you." My kids learned what that meant as we ate our tenth lasagna! Never underestimate the relief that a frozen meal can offer a tired family. Almost anyone can provide a simple meal to someone in need. Another friend offered to clean my house. I regret that I didn't take her up on it. I had way too much pride to let someone clean my bathrooms and kitchen. She even offered to do laundry. I couldn't bear to let someone see my dirty laundry piles. Now I kick myself when I think of passing up such help. I probably robbed my dear friend of the joy of helping out as well. What's the best part of the twin friend? She's right where you are and knows what you need most. She knew I had loads and loads of laundry, as well as dirty bathtubs. I am ashamed of myself for not accepting her gift. Swallow your pride, thank God for your twin friends, and let them help you. I'm relieved to read in Galatians 6:2 (NKJV) where Paul says to "bear one another's burdens and so fulfill the law of Christ." Aren't dinners, piles of dirty clothes, exhaustion, dirty bathrooms, unkempt kitchens, and groceries a burden when you have a newborn? Let your friends bear your burdens and be obedient to Christ! One of the hardest things for women to do is to accept help. I think we are forcing friends to miss out on blessings when we won't let them love us.

The next type of friend discussed was the "sparkler friend." This person is high intensity as well as high maintenance. They can get the joy out of any situation. These people remember to celebrate and, boy, do they know how. They go all out and give everything 100%. They tend to blow everything out of proportion and have a flare for the dramatic. They are the last people to call in a crisis, but they are good grievers. These friends are fun to play with and bring sparkles to our most ordinary days. I am so thankful to God that he kept my sparkler friends far away from me when I was in crisis. But they were wonderful to have around as I started to breathe again. One friend in particular kept after me about exercising and getting out of the house. Another sparkler was upset with me for quitting some of my activities. Both of these friends were convinced I'd heal if I'd just get back into activities and fill up my social calendar. I prayed that God would take them away from me and he did. They backed off, which was totally out of character; I know God had his hand in that. One more lady that I consider a sparkler friend was wonderful to pray with when I couldn't find the words to say. She would pray the most beautiful prayers to God on my behalf. Her joy kept a little light burning in my darkness. God delicately brought the sparklers I needed at exactly the time I needed them.

The third type of friend is the "rock friend." This is the most seasoned mother, usually the oldest of your support system. This is the woman whom you ask, "How fast can you get here?" You can call her day or night and she can solve your problems. Sometimes this friend attempts to solve things before you even ask. She can take over because she knows what needs to be done in almost any situation. My rock friend lives at least a thousand miles away in the heart of Texas. I can call her whenever I need a mother to listen to me who *isn't* my mother. She treats me like a daughter, but we have a different relationship than my mother and I do. I enjoy getting her advice even when we don't see eye to eye. I love hearing how she had similar problems with her kids decades ago. I feel stronger after talking to her. She makes me realize that I can get through this. Today is not the worst day. Tomorrow will be okay, because God is still going to be there. I know that while I was going through my PPD she was praying for me. Even when she didn't know very much about what was happening to me, I know she was praying. God has placed a burden on her heart to pray for our family. I have no reason to believe that she'll stop anytime soon. She prays for me, my husband, and each one of my children. It makes me feel so loved by God that he would meet that need for our family. If you don't have a person praying for you and your family by name, I am begging you to go find that person. God wants that for you. I'm convinced that my life is much better off with my friend interceding for us! Philemon 7 (NIV) says, "Your love has given me great joy and encouragement, because you, brother, have refreshed the hearts of the saints." My dear friend has taught me that only God can give us true joy and encouragement, so why not ask him for it? During the hardest times of my life she has been my rock. The best part about her is that she's always pointed me to the true rock, Jesus.

Another type of friend in our lives is the "been there friend." This is typically an older woman, in some cases our own mothers. They remind us that everything is going to work out and be just fine. As my own mother says, "This too shall pass." I don't know how that helps when you're in the middle of a crisis, but I try to remember it nonetheless. These friends reassure us that things will get better. It's easy to spend a lot of time venting with these people. They are easy to talk to and are extremely sympathetic. We have to be careful not to run over these friends. We tend to run over them like doormats because they are such good listeners. At the beginning of my nightmare with PPD, I was terrified to confide in anyone. Then something huge happened for me. One night a woman I barely knew from Bible study asked me the dreaded question, "Do you have the baby blues?" Now you already know my feelings about these awful words, but for some reason they didn't bother me. I felt like hugging her and never letting go. It was as if she saw me and knew me like no one else could. I knew then and there that someone real had been through some of what I had. I didn't need to know her story, and she didn't need to know mine. We had an unspoken understanding of each other's pain. All my other friends needed explanations and clarification. She just knew by looking at me what was happening. I was so grateful to God that this woman gave me her time and attention. Our paths didn't cross too often during my crisis months, but God gave me her just when I needed her most.

During my illness our interim pastor preached on "coming alongside" people during their various experiences in life. More often than not, people just need someone to physically be there with them during tough times. Words don't always do much good. Usually we can't do all that much to help. But we can use our own experiences to comfort others.

> "Praise be to the God and Father of our Lord Jesus Christ, the Father of compassion and the God of all comfort, who comforts us in all our troubles, so that we can comfort those in any trouble with the comfort we ourselves have received from God."
> (2 Corinthians 1:3–4, NIV)

Sometimes God can use our horrible life experiences to help others down the road. My friend had been through an awful time with PPD and could comfort me with the fact that she was over the illness. When you are in the middle of such an intense experience, you can't imagine any end in sight. Just the fact that she was standing there in front of me, completely free of this depression, gave me a glimmer of hope. It made me seek help. I knew I had a chance. Thank God for my "been there" friend! Most women who suffer from PPD don't get the help they need. I believe that this woman was placed in my life by God to get me to seek help. She couldn't help me with all my psychological or physical needs, but she showed concern and compassion that made all the difference in the world. Now that I am on the other side of my illness, I look forward to meeting the women God has prepared for me to comfort. I know without a shadow of a doubt that I experienced these horrible circumstances for a wonderful purpose. I cannot wait to walk alongside someone and encourage them during their struggle with PPD. God can and will bring good out of my pain and suffering.

The next type of friend is known as the "challenging one." These aren't friends that we need, but they tend to stick with us. They don't go away easily. These friends can be toxic. Life has limits, and these gals push those constantly. They suck up our time and energy, not to mention our joy. If people around you make you feel worse about yourself and the world around you, then you should lovingly walk away from them. These clingy, needy friends are not the ones you need in a crisis. I have recently had only one such clingy friend. She told me that if I wouldn't be her best friend and commit to calling her every day, then she didn't want to have anything to do with me. Let's just say I don't currently have that person in my life. I feel no need to revert back to the good old junior high drama. I do, however, have another generally challenging friend. She is quite obnoxious to be honest. She knows everything and tells everyone what to do. She is the classic Type A bossy girl that no one could stand in elementary school. I praise God that he answered my prayers and kept her away from my house for a period of time. I couldn't have coped with her telling me to snap out of it and to get back to my life. God really shielded me from challenging friends during my PPD. Don't get me wrong. I do believe these friends are in our lives for a reason. God can use us to minister to them, and I believe he wants us to. But when we are in a crisis, these are friends to shy away from at all costs.

The last kind of friend that Allie Pleiter talked about was the "best-ever girlfriend." This friend is a one of a kind gem. She is not replaceable. You grieve when this friend is gone. You can just go to their house at the drop of a hat. You can swimsuit shop together. You can tell each other what size you wear and how much you weigh. She probably knows the first boy you kissed. I've had so much change in my life that I'm not sure I've ever made the time investment it takes to nurture such a friendship. At times I thought I had best-ever friends, but it turns out I liked them a whole lot more than they liked me. I have two precious friends that were going to visit me in the psych unit. Those poor women had no idea what they were getting involved with. Thank goodness I was discharged from the hospital before they could see the circus. But just knowing they would have come made me feel overwhelmed with love and humility. I received phone calls from them while I was in the psychiatric unit. Just hearing their voices was like breathing fresh air. Don't underestimate the power of a phone call. I also have another friend who helped with my kids and listened to my jibber jabber month after month. She never judged me or questioned me. She just listened. I felt so much support from her. Maybe one day we'll even swimsuit shop together. I am so grateful for the best-ever friend that God is working on just for me.

Allie concluded her session with a few reminders of how to make friends. First, God cares, so ask him about your friendships. Do you want friends? Do you need certain kinds of friends? Are you needing guidance in the area of challenging friends? Second, our friendships need maintenance. We have to be willing to put in the time to make our relationships flourish and grow. Third, we need to practice the art of forgiveness. We are all human and make mistakes along the way. In order for friendships to survive, we have to forgive each other. Lastly, if we don't have the important types of friends that we need in various situations, Christ can fill the void. Jesus can fill in every one of the gaps. He can be with us in a way that no person can ever be. Even my husband, who is my best-ever friend, cannot meet the deepest needs of my life. Only Christ can accomplish that.

Why all this talk about friends in the middle of a serious topic like postpartum depression? I know that God gave me people for every single thing I needed during my battle with PPD. I needed physical people to see and to hold me. I needed help with accomplishing daily tasks

The Lifter of My Head

such as food and laundry. I am sure that God sent me those people. He sent me friends that I didn't even know I needed. If it were not for the people God sent me, I don't know what would've become of me. I am so grateful for the friends God handpicked for me. I am also glad for the pruning he did of my relationships. In the months before I had the baby, I lost two significant friends. I remember being devastated at the loss of them. It was as if one day they just disappeared off the face of the planet. I have no idea what I did or what happened to change our relationships. I left messages and rang doorbells but they were just gone. It was as if we were never friends to start with. I was crushed, because I thought we were so close, but I was just so wrong. Now, in hindsight, I am so grateful that I lost these friends before I went through my PPD. It would've crushed me to have to deal with their apathy at such a time. I will be forever grateful that God showed me who my genuine friends were before the storm hit.

The last friend I would like to examine is one that I've added to Allie's list. It's what I like to call the "holier-than-thou" type. Sometimes these people can camouflage themselves fairly well. It is only when tough times come that you see their true colors. Some people don't even know they have such an offensive attitude. When I had depression after my first child, I experienced this silly attitude first hand. I was ignorant of PPD, and my obstetrician treated me as if I was an idiot. He gave me a very low dose of antidepressant and said literally, "Get over it, it's just a baby. Just quit crying already. You'll feel better if you go home and have sex." I'm not kidding you, that's what he said! I had no reason not to not trust him, so I believed I could just "get over" my depression. It lasted a long time, and I suffered terribly.

When my daughter was about nine months old, I went back to work. I was overwhelmed with stress, guilt, and crazy hormones; most days I didn't know which end was up. I started fantasizing about running my car off the road as I was commuting to work. Every day I would hit the same spot in the highway and have a picture in my mind of the car crashing. My heart would pound and I would break into a sweat. I was scared of my thoughts. I had no idea what was happening to me. I decided one Sunday night after the church service to confide in someone I deeply trusted. I shared with her as much as I thought I could, sugarcoating the whole story. In my desperation I still wanted to appear all put together and "Christian." Her reaction blew me away. Her first words were in the form of a devastating question, "Have you been spending time in prayer and reading your Bible?" I didn't know much about PPD at the time, but I seriously doubted it had much to do with my spiritual health. Her reaction clearly showed me that she didn't know anything about PPD. It also made me feel extreme shame concerning my illness. Words can hurt or heal a spirit. The Bible says, "The tongue has the power of life and death..." (Proverbs 18:21, NIV). Her reaction had the potential to make or break our relationship. I have forgiven her, but her attitude and comment have left a scar on my heart. I have since realized that controlling our words is the truest expression of wisdom. I'm confident that this woman was holier than me in that she spent hours in prayer and Bible study, while I was hobbling along day to day in my spiritual walk. I'll never doubt that she's "better" than me, but I'm not competing any more. I've learned that comparing myself to others is just a waste of precious time and energy. God wants us to know him and spend time with him. I don't believe he has a timer set to see how long we read our Bibles and pray. I have asked God many times to give me the desire to know him more. He's answered my prayer every time. Now I earnestly pray that I'll never treat someone like I am better than them spiritually. What a silly concept.

After my daughter, our first child, was born, I pleaded with God to make me well. One day he did. In the meantime I learned a lot about PPD and even more about the impact of our words on people. First, you shouldn't talk about things you don't understand. I have an acquaintance that broke her leg last year. Can you imagine me asking her during that time if she was reading her Bible and praying enough? Somehow her leg would've been spared had she been closer to God? That's ridiculous! But as Christians we tend to judge things we don't understand. If things are uncomfortable for us then they must be related to sin. In general, mental illness of any kind is seen in the Christian world as a character flaw. Most people don't begin to understand mental illness, so it's just easier to judge it and give out worthless and uninformed advice. I think it's best if we just listen and learn about things before we talk about them. My husband told me recently, "People see the world through their own experiences. That's all they have." It's excruciating to try to break through the barrier of ignorance, especially when it's coupled with criticism. The second thing I learned was if you can't say something nice don't say anything at all. As a child I didn't really grasp the power of that, now I do. Let's look at the Scriptures for more wisdom concerning nice words. "A gentle answer turns away wrath, but a harsh word stirs up anger." (Proverbs 15:1, NIV) "Watch your words and hold your tongue, you'll save yourself a lot of grief." (Proverbs 21:23, Msg) "Therefore encourage one another and build each other up..." (1 Thessalonians 5:11a, NIV) Only kind words can build up others. The third thing about words that I learned was from a recent sermon. Our pastor preached a series of sermons about "street wisdom" from Proverbs. Naturally, we spent time evaluating our behavior, especially our words. I discovered that it is very Christian to keep our mouths shut. I've always had a lot to say about everything, so this was particularly hard for me to hear. Over the years God has taught me how to keep my mouth shut and still be happy. "When words are many, sin is not absent, but he who holds his tongue is wise." (Proverbs 10:19, NIV) Proverbs 17:27–28 (NIV) makes a great point: "A man of knowledge uses words with restraint, and a man of understanding is even-tempered. Even a fool is thought wise if he keeps silent, and discerning if he holds his tongue."

In conclusion, God has taught me so much about the gift of friendship through my illness. Although he has most recently blessed me with incredibly genuine and loving friends, he's previously blessed me even during times of no friends. I've learned that Jesus is my best friend. I've gained wisdom on how to come alongside others in Christian fellowship. I've discovered a secret to service: just do it. I've learned to listen better and love better by keeping my mouth shut. I've discovered that my circle of influence takes priority over my circle of concern. I've learned to accept kindness and say thank you. I don't know if I'll be able to adequately thank all the people God has given me during my PPD experience. I figure God will just bless those who have been faithful to him, who have loved me when I needed it most. I believe if I just give God the glory by sharing who and what he's provided for me, then my friends will be blessed immeasurably by him.

Food for thought
"If you can't feed 100 people, then just feed one."
— Mother Theresa

"Grant that I may not so much seek to be consoled as to console; to be understood as to understand; to be loved as to love; for it is in giving that we receive, it is in pardoning that we are pardoned, and it is in dying that we are born to eternal life."
—St. Francis of Assissi.

"Happiness is a perfume you cannot pour on others without getting a few drops on yourself."
—Euripides, ancient Greek playwright

Healthcare Professionals God Used

"Come to me, all you who are weary and burdened, and I will give you rest." (Matthew 11:28, NIV)

"And my God will meet all your needs according to his glorious riches in Christ Jesus." (Philippians 4:19, NIV)

When I first felt my illness taking over, I resisted seeking professional care. I repeatedly denied that I was sick. I was inclined to trust my instincts—that I would heal given enough time and rest. I also knew that I was simply fooling myself. It was exhausting to attempt to keep up the charade with others and practically impossible with myself. Lying to yourself is a tough and time-consuming task. Once I decided to contact my obstetrician, I thought I would stop the pretending. But when I got to my appointment with him, I sugarcoated most of what I shared. I had multiple opportunities to reach out to someone with the truth, but I didn't. Maybe I was scared of the truth, the reality that I was getting progressively worse by the day. I'm confident that I had no clue what was yet to come, or I might have skipped the whole act with my doctor. Within six weeks I tried to make a follow-up appointment and ended up in the emergency room instead. I tell you this because if you're anything like me, you don't always seek the help you need. Somewhere in our formative years it was impressed upon us to help ourselves or worse yet, "God helps those who help themselves." I saw admitting that I needed help as a sign of weakness, a fruit of my failure as a new mother. I am also sharing this with you so that you'll know of the professional help that's out there. Before I was sick, I had no idea that most of the following healthcare and information existed. Like Dr. Phil McGraw says, "You can't change what you don't acknowledge." Let's move forward, acknowledging that we need help, and there is a load of it out there for the taking.

First and foremost, if you recognize any symptoms of postpartum depression, contact your obstetrician. I would highly recommend seeing the doctor you saw during your pregnancy if at all possible. I would also strongly recommend that you avoid seeing your family practice doctor. Your symptoms might be mild and may not require much intervention, but a family practice doctor is limited in knowledge about severe postpartum depression. More than likely you will be referred to an obstetrician or psychologist anyway. Why waste precious time running around to appointments when you need to get well? My obstetrician did my initial assessment and prescribed me an antidepressant. I was immediately enrolled in a program through my insurance company called "On Your Way." I received newsletters every once in awhile, encouraging me as I healed. The most interesting part was that the people who put the newsletter together really understood about my illness. It brought me so much comfort that my illness was running its course. My doctor couldn't talk to me every week, but he knew the importance of getting valuable literature in my hands. There were several people in my doctor's office who played an integral part in my care. Don't underestimate the words of support that can come from a receptionist or registered nurse. My obstetrician's nurse treated me as if I were her own daughter. She was genuinely concerned about my well-being. I'll not soon forget the woman who answered the phone the day I tried to make a follow-up appointment. She regretted that I couldn't get an appointment that day, but insisted I see someone in family practice. I urged her to believe me that family practice wouldn't cut it. She transferred me to someone in triage, sensing the urgency of my call. The triage nurse on the other end of the phone had a familiar voice. After a few sentences, I recognized her as the first person I'd ever spoken with in that office. She was the first nurse I met with when I had discovered I was pregnant. She had done my required nutrition visit. She told me how to best exercise and eat to keep me and the baby healthy. We talked about prenatal vitamins and avoiding caffeine, things of that nature. It thrilled me to hear a familiar voice. Even better—she remembered me. I know that God put her on that phone on that day with me. She gave me a sense of safety and comfort. She also knew that I was fond of my obstetrician's nurse. She allowed me to speak with her for a few minutes. This may seem like a huge exaggeration to you, but I firmly believe that speaking with those two women that day may have saved my life. I don't know if I was ever seriously suicidal, but I do know I considered it for a short time. Hearing their reassurances was enough for me to get to the bottom of the mess I was in, so that I could get out of it. My experience was atypical—that's why I testify that God had his mighty hand in it. I've never had a medical doctor, a receptionist, and a few RNs who were that concerned about me. They worked together to get me to the help I needed.

My next piece of advice is to listen to your obstetrician, or any doctor for that matter, even if it seems scary. I realize there are nutty doctors out there, so use your judgment. I also know that many Christians think you shouldn't see doctors when you are sick. Hopefully, you can use the brain God gave you and do what is right. I bring this up, because my obstetrician's advice terrified me. I was told, via the RN, that I needed to get to the emergency room as soon as possible. They wanted to know when I'd be leaving and what exact time I thought I would arrive. My RN even contacted my husband for me so I could focus on getting someone to watch the kids and get to the hospital. I had no understanding whatsoever about what would transpire at the hospital. I stepped out in faith that my obstetrician knew what was best for me. I trusted that God gave us a good rapport for a reason. I was out of my mind and frightened beyond my wildest imagination. But, the important thing is that I went to the hospital.

The next phase of my care began in the emergency room and then shifted to the behavioral health unit. I share this part of my story with you so that you won't be scared like I was. If you ever reach the point of losing your mind, let the experts help you. I went into the psychiatric unit almost kicking and screaming. I was out of control with panic and fear. Part of the problem was my illness; the other part was the fear of the unknown. The first person I recall helping me in the emergency room was the needs–assessment person. She had to determine if I was in crisis and then what level of care I needed. In all honesty, she was the first person who ever heard my whole life story without any filtering. She learned of the pain of my childhood and crushing baggage of my teen years. She knew the good, the bad, and ultimately the ugly. She knew more details of my postpartum depression than anyone else. I was at a point of desperation and simply trusted her with everything. I ended up in the psychiatric unit, which is still a puzzle to me, but I trusted this woman with my life. Knowing what I do now, I still would have shared all that I did, even though it cost me a few days without my family. I needed time to rest, space away from my responsibilities. I needed to confide in trustworthy professionals. My stay in the hospital met all those needs. I thank God for the needs-assessment woman. She knew I needed help. I'm not sure I like how every detail was handled, but in the end, I got to the next stage of help that I needed.

I was such a mess by the time I got to the psychiatric unit, that quite a few details are foggy in my memory. Everyone wore name badges, bearing titles I'd never heard of. I kept seeing B.H.A. and B.H. Specialist, as well as social worker variations. I talked to a lot of different people and didn't have a clue who was going to help me next. I spent a full night not sure of who was there to help me and who might try to kill me. The next morning, I quickly found a woman who would be my God-send. I knew immediately that she was there for me. I went to group therapy sessions and she was there. When she wasn't leading sessions, she was in the hall ready to talk to me. I took full advantage of every opportunity that I had to speak with her. I asked dozens of questions. She connected me with someone who seemed to be a doctor of sorts. Between the two of them, I felt I always had someone on my side. They wasted no time in getting to the bottom of what was happening to me. I felt reassured as the doctor explained to me that I didn't do anything wrong, that I couldn't have planned for this. He said it could have happened even if I had previously told my obstetrician every detail of my symptoms. I felt a precious relationship develop instantly with both of these healthcare professionals. I knew in months to come I would give thanks to God for bringing me to them. I believed they would let me go home when I was ready; I no longer feared staying in the hospital with all the other "crazy" people. I can joke about that term now because I've been there. We were all out of our minds at that time, and that can create a bizarre atmosphere. We were kindred spirits in some weird sense. It wasn't much like *Girl Interrupted* with Angelina Jolie. It wasn't at all like *One Flew Over the Cuckoo's Nest* with Jack Nicholson. It was more like *The Breakfast Club* with lots of Judd Nelsons trying to have successful therapy sessions with all the Ally Sheedys. That's where the different staff members came into the picture. They gave everyone a sense of normalcy and dignity. We were treated like hurting people, not crazy patients. Once I accepted my temporary fate, I trusted God to give me the best care through these people. I did everything they told me to. I gave my therapy sessions one hundred percent. I answered all their questions and took all my medicine. I thank God that he gave me full confidence that these people knew what they were doing. Because of their respect, I was able to openly discuss my illness with the on–call psychiatrist.

I waited for what seemed like an eternity to speak with the hospital's psychiatrist. One full day is like a lifetime when you are locked in a building with no escape. The doctor was my ticket out and I was ready for her. I had no idea what to expect. After a few minutes of conversation, she told me I was going home. That's when I really dove in and told her what was going on in my mind. As soon as I knew she would let me go home, I felt free to express my fears, not only about the psychiatric unit, but about my future as a mentally ill mom. She promised me that this hospital stay was temporary. She assured me that if I would follow her recommendations concerning my treatment, I would soon be one hundred percent myself again. She didn't sugarcoat a thing. She said I would need intensive therapy sessions and months of a medication regimen. Because she filtered nothing with me, I was able to keep being totally honest and open with her. She had me well-prepared for the next phase of my healing: outpatient care.

I was assigned a social worker who contacted me a few times a week to check on me. There was nothing innately personal about our conversations, but I felt accountable to her. I felt such relief when she would call. Just hearing her voice made me feel like someone still cared, even though the crisis had passed. In the big picture, she played a seemingly small role. It's uncanny how her voice lifted my spirits. I was fully aware that I was just a case of hers, but it didn't matter. I felt special and cared for. Only the love of God can make you feel that way, so I believe that God was using that insignificant relationship to do big things to boost my spirit. I am grateful that God gave me the strength to keep answering her calls, and that she loved her job. She called me one day, early in the week after I'd been discharged from the hospital. She set up an appointment for me to meet with a psychologist. At that point, I wasn't too fired up about it, but I didn't have a thing to lose.

My gut instinct, while standing in the psychologist's office, waiting to be addressed by the receptionist, was to run. I was prepared to flee. I hated standing in that place with a fiery passion. I had come full circle and was terrified to admit anything about my illness. All over again, I was in denial. I was quite paranoid. If I shared the wrong information, I realized that this person had the power to put me back in the hospital. She could make the recommendation and that would be the end of my freedom, again. It took a long time for me to trust this person. I am, unfortunately, one of those people who trusts anyone. I am easily duped, easily hurt. But this relationship was different. From the beginning, our relationship was forcefully created because I was sick. I wasn't in crisis anymore, so it annoyed me to talk to this person about my daily struggles. I initially resisted working through my issues with her. I just wanted to use my "get out of jail free" card with her and be on my way. Therapy sessions in the hospital were a necessary evil. Dreading a *weekly* therapy session was unbearable. I felt horrible every day, just waiting to talk about my bad things going on. I didn't get the feeling that she knew a whole lot about postpartum depression. That discouraged me from sharing at first. As I worked through my issues and initial disappointment with my therapist, I gave in and started trusting her instincts about my illness. I began to see that she knew me like a book. She perceived my personality. She noticed how I communicated. She saw what various traumas had done to me, how my childhood formed the adult sitting in her office, how love lost had grieved me, how apathy in others had scarred me. She was the first person to ever verbalize to me that she really did get it. I heard Dr. Phil say once on his talk show, something to this effect, "We cannot truly heal from our life's scars unless someone sees us and understands what we've experienced." For most of us, we need the acknowledgment that what we went through was real and that it had a huge impact on us. As we dissected my life with PPD, I learned to "ride it out" as my therapist suggested. She said I should let my illness run its natural course and quit fighting it. I quit trying to fix everything at once. I learned to deal with one problem at a time. As my depression and anxiety subsided, we dealt with a lifetime of hurts. I regret that we didn't get to all of them, but frankly I was tired of talking. I am sharing a lot about my therapy because I don't know how I would have healed without it. God provided this valuable resource to me even when I didn't want it. He knew what I needed. I needed information and support. But I also needed a face to see every week. I needed someone that knew me inside and out. He gave my therapist great insight. I know she's brilliant, but I also believe God had his hand in my therapy sessions. For months I struggled to work through my agonizing therapy. I feel that without God's hand in the process, I would still be in weekly sessions. I thank God for the precious time that I spent getting help from this woman. Most of what we talked about is a blur to me now. (That would not come as a surprise to my therapist; she says that's part of my personality.) But I am thankful for the skills she taught me for coping with my illness.

I am grateful for the opportunity to talk through some old issues as well. My time spent in that office was excruciating but necessary for an even deeper healing of my soul. For decades I had carried some huge baggage. When I left that office for what I knew would be the last time, I left all that mess behind me. I left years worth of pain and never looked back. I discovered through many sessions and much prayer that God loved me enough for me to move on. I didn't have to keep beating myself up and asking why about the various circumstances of my life. My therapy helped me to clearly see that I deserved more out of my life than pain. My therapist helped to restore my self-esteem and spirit. She urged me to immerse myself in Scripture and surround myself with my Christian girlfriends. She saw me evolve from a complete mess, straight from the psychiatric unit, to a confident woman, ready to see my illness through to the end.

God used numerous and various healthcare professionals to bring about my healing. Did he need to use them? No. Was I glad he did? Yes. God can choose to make us well without using anyone, but I think he likes using people. I learned a lot from the process of healing. If God had chosen to wipe out my sickness, I would have missed out on a lot of relationships with extraordinary people. Most of them saw at least a part of my recuperation. It must be a blessing to those workers to see cases of great success with mental illness. Many of them got to see how I trusted God to use them to help me. It was a fascinating miracle that God worked in my life. He worked out so many details in my healthcare. He brought me the people that best suited me. I am not ashamed to admit that I needed help, and a lot of it. I am stunned at how God executed his plan of healing in my fragile life. If he can heal me, I know he can heal you. Don't be afraid to seek help. God wants us to live whole and holy lives. He wants good things for his children, so why don't you ask him? Jesus reassures us, "If you, then, though you are evil, know how to give good gifts to your children, how much more will your Father in heaven give good gifts to those who ask him!" (Matthew 7:11, NIV). You could be surprised who and what he might use. Don't be hesitant when he uses unconventional methods to bring about your wholeness. He delights in our living life victoriously and then giving him the credit. It's almost as if he planned it that way.

Food for thought:
"The best way to find yourself, is to lose yourself in the service of others."

—Ghandi

"You have not lived until you have done something for someone who can never repay you."

—Anonymous

"God has given us two hands, one to receive with and the other to give with."

—Billy Graham, Evangelist

The Lifter of My Head

"But you are a shield around me, O Lord; you bestow glory on me and lift up my head. To the Lord I cry aloud and he answers me from his holy hill...I lie down and sleep; I wake again, because the Lord sustains me." (Psalm 3:3–5, NIV)

"I waited patiently for the Lord to help me, and he turned to me and heard my cry. He lifted me out of the pit of despair, out of the mud and the mire. He set my feet on solid ground and steadied me as I walked along." (Psalm 40:1–2, NLT)

Reading God's word and praying to him are the perfect remedy to any of life's ailments. God reveals himself to us through his word. You can feel his support and unconditional love in his words. I sensed his love supporting me and lifting me up as I talked to him. As others prayed for me, I felt God lifting me up out of my pit of depression. God didn't create us to be depressed. He created us to live life abundantly. I found abundant life anew as I searched his word and prayed to him.

When I was in college, we often sang a simple chorus as a prayer to close church services. "Thou, oh Lord, art a shield about me. You're my glory, you're the lifter of my head. Alleluia. Alleluia. Alleluia. You're the lifter of my head." Those simple words have stirred my heart in a brand new way. They have brought me much relief on days I saw no hope. I genuinely felt like God literally lifted my head up on many days. Some days, he had to continuously hold it up for me. A multitude of circumstances lead people to hang their heads in defeat or shame. I've been there and I bet you have, too. Postpartum depression left me feeling completely deflated. It just knocked the life out of me. Each and every day, God gave me a fresh start, a renewed perspective, a lifted head. Over and over again, I would hang my head in defeat and fear. I had to repeatedly ask him for support. I had to spend time in his word. It became nourishment to me. I held on to the comforting words I read. I read the Bible as if God wrote it for just little, old me. It became intensely personal. He met my needs every single day. I saw his faithfulness to me and it led me to a cycle of belief and trust. The more I saw him do, the more I believed and trusted in him. In turn, he would show more of his love and power in my life. I would then believe and trust in him more. It was a beautiful pattern. You might be wondering exactly how he did that. I had three things going for me that I know God provided: great health care, faithful Christian friends praying for me, and my Bible to read. I've already told you about my great friends and healthcare professionals. I now want to share with you how Bible study and prayer sustained me.

 I struggled to read my Bible. I knew I had to do it, but it was mentally painful. I didn't dare attempt any type of structured Bible study. My mind was blurry, my thoughts too fragmented. God was gracious to me in my lack of discipline. I could only muster the strength to read snippets of Scripture. I needed quick access to Scriptures that were particularly meaningful. Fortunately, I had a system already in place. As a young child, I watched my oldest brother write Bible verses on index cards. He stored them in a plastic, tan container on his desk. Sometimes he let me watch him write his Bible verses and practice memorizing them. I was fascinated by his collection of white, 4x6 index cards. As soon as I was old enough to write, I wrote Bible verses on index cards. I had a hideous, avocado green, recipe box that my mother gave me. I used it for decades to guard my treasure of Scripture. To this day, I use index cards to quickly review some of my favorites. During my illness, I nearly wore out my cards. I would like to share the Scriptures that God kept placing on my heart. Many of these verses have been dear to me for years. However, they have become permanent fixtures on my heart this last year. I have organized them according to pertinent questions. I hope and pray that God will breathe a special life into these, just for you.

Will I ever overcome this illness?

> "...in all these things we are more than conquerors through him who loved us. For I am convinced that neither death nor life, neither angels nor demons, neither the present nor the future, nor any powers, neither height nor depth, nor anything else in all creation, will be able to separate us from the love of God that is in Christ Jesus our Lord." (Romans 8:37–39, NIV)

Where can I go for help?

"...Let the beloved of the LORD rest secure in him, for he shields him all day long, and the one the LORD loves rests between his shoulders." (Deuteronomy 33:12, NIV)

"The LORD is a refuge for the oppressed, a stronghold in times of trouble. Those who know your name will trust in you, LORD, for you have never forsaken those who seek you." (Psalm 9:9–10, NIV)

"The Lord is my light and my salvation—whom shall I fear? The Lord is the stronghold of my life—of whom shall I be afraid? For in the day of trouble he will keep me safe in his dwelling; he will hide me in the shelter of his tabernacle and set me high upon a rock. Then my head will be exalted..." (Psalm 27:1; 5; 6a, NIV)

"Surely God is my help; the Lord is the one who sustains me." (Psalm 54:4, NIV)

"Truly my soul silently waits for God; from him comes my salvation; he is my defense; I shall not be greatly moved." (Psalm 62:1–2, NKJV)

"On my bed I remember you; I think of you through the watches of the night. Because you are my help, I sing in the shadow of your wings." (Psalm 63:6–7, NIV)

"For I am the LORD, your God, who takes hold of your right hand and says to you, Do not fear; I will help you." (Isaiah 41:13, NIV)

Does God have the power to help me?

"...Nothing can hinder the LORD from saving, whether by many or few." (I Samuel 14:6, NIV)

"You give me your shield of victory, and your right hand sustains me; you stoop down to make me great." (Psalm 18:35, NIV)

"Your ways, O God, are holy. What god is so great as our God? You are the God who performs miracles; you display your power among the peoples." (Psalm 77:13–14, NIV)

"You answer us with awesome deeds of righteousness, O God our Savior..." (Psalm 65: 5, NIV)

"Ah, Sovereign LORD, you have made the heavens and the earth by your great power and outstretched arm. Nothing is too hard for you." (Jeremiah 32:17, NIV)

"His divine power has given us everything we need for life and godliness through the knowledge of him..." (2 Peter 1:3, NIV)

Can God give me peace?

"The Lord gives strength to his people; the Lord blesses his people with peace." (Psalm 29:11, NIV)

"When you lie down, you will not be afraid; when you lie down, your sleep will be sweet. For the Lord will be your confidence..." (Proverbs 3:24; 26, NIV)

"'Though the mountains be shaken and the hills be removed, yet my unfailing love for you will not be shaken nor my covenant of peace be removed,' says the Lord, who has compassion on you." (Isaiah 54:10, NIV)

"And he (Jesus) will be their peace." (Micah 5:5, NIV)

Does God love me, even when I'm sick?

"He reached down from on high and took hold of me; he drew me out of deep waters. He brought me out into a spacious place; he rescued me because he delighted in me." (Psalm 18:16; 19, NIV)

"You restored me to health and let me live. Surely it was for my benefit that I suffered such anguish." (Isaiah 38:16b-17a, NIV)

"The LORD will guide you always; he will satisfy your needs in a sun-scorched land and will strengthen your frame. You will be like a well-watered garden, like a spring whose waters never fail. Your people will rebuild the ancient ruins and will raise up the age-old foundations; you will be called Repairer of Broken Walls, Restorer of Streets with Dwellings." (Isaiah 58:11–12, NIV)

"The LORD your God is with you, he is mighty to save. He will take great delight in you, he will quiet you with his love, he will rejoice over you with singing." (Zephaniah 3:17, NIV)

"…Jesus said, 'It is not the healthy who need a doctor, but the sick.'" (Matthew 9:12, NIV)

"Jesus went through all the towns and villages, teaching in their synagogues, preaching the good news of the kingdom and healing every disease and sickness." (Matthew 9:35, NIV)

Will God stick it out with me?

"Thus far has the LORD helped us." (1 Samuel 7:12b, NIV)

"Because of the LORD's great love we are not consumed, for his compassions never fail. They are new every morning; great is your faithfulness." (Lamentations 3:22–23, NIV)

"O LORD God Almighty, who is like you? You are mighty, O LORD, and your faithfulness surrounds you." (Psalm 89:8, NIV)

"Do you not know? Have you not heard? The LORD is the everlasting God, the Creator of the ends of the earth. He will not grow tired or weary, and his understanding no one can fathom. He gives strength to the weary and increases the power of the weak." (Isaiah 40:28–29, NIV)

"Listen to me, O house of Jacob, all you who remain in the house of Israel, you whom I have upheld since you were conceived, and have carried since your birth. Even to your old age and gray hairs I am he, I am he who will sustain you. I have made you and I will carry you; I will sustain you and I will rescue you." (Isaiah 46:3–4, NIV)

Does God truly see and hear me?

"I will be glad and rejoice in your love, for you saw my affliction and knew the anguish of my soul. You have not handed me over to my enemy but have set my feet in a spacious place." (Psalm 31:7–8, NIV)

"Can a mother forget the baby at her breast and have no compassion on the child she has borne? Though she may forget, I will not forget you! See, I have engraved you on the palms of my hands..." (Isaiah 49:15–16, NIV)

"I waited patiently for the LORD; he turned to me and heard my cry. He lifted me out of the slimy pit, out of the mud and mire; he set my feet on a rock and gave me a firm place to stand." (Psalm 40:1–2, NIV)

"Call to me and I will answer you. I'll tell you marvelous and wondrous things that you could never figure out on your own." (Jeremiah 33:3, Msg)

What does God expect of me?

"My tears have been my food day and night. Why are you downcast, O my soul? Why so disturbed within me? Put your hope in God, for I will yet praise him, my Savior and my God." (Psalm 42:3,5, NIV)

"Write down for the coming generation what the Lord has done so that people not yet born will praise him." (Psalm 102:18, TEV)

"Publish his glorious deeds among the nations. Tell everyone about the amazing things he does." (Psalm 96:3, NLT)

"I don't want your sacrifices, I want your love! I don't want your offerings—I want you to know me." (Hosea 6:6, TLB)

"He has showed you, O man, what is good. And what does the Lord require of you? To act justly and to love mercy and to walk humbly with your God." (Micah 6:8, NIV)

"And without faith it is impossible to please God, because anyone who comes to him must believe that he exists and that he rewards those who earnestly seek him." (Hebrews 11:6, NIV)

How will life ever get back to normal?

"The Spirit of the Sovereign Lord is on me (Jesus), because the Lord has anointed me to preach good news to the poor. He has sent me to bind up the brokenhearted, to proclaim freedom for the captives and release from darkness for the prisoners, to proclaim the year of the Lord's favor and the day of vengeance of our God, to comfort all who mourn, and provide for those who grieve in Zion—to bestow on them a crown of beauty instead of ashes, the oil of gladness instead of mourning, and a garment of praise instead a spirit of despair. They will be called oaks of righteousness, a planting of the Lord for the display of his splendor. They will rebuild the ancient ruins and restore the places long devastated; they will renew the ruined cities that have been devastated for generations." (Isaiah 61:1–4, NIV)

"I am still confident of this; I will see the goodness of the Lord in the land of the living." (Psalm 27:13, NIV)

"I am the LORD your God, who brought you up out of Egypt. Open wide your mouth and I will fill it." (Psalm 81:10, NIV)

"For I know the plans I have for you," declares the LORD, "plans to prosper you and not to harm you, plans to give you hope and a future. Then you will call upon me and come and pray to me, and I will listen to you. You will seek me and find me when you seek me with all your heart. I will be found by you," declares the LORD." (Jeremiah 29:11–14, NIV)

"Jesus looked at them and said, 'With man this is impossible, but with God all things are possible.'" (Matthew 19:26, NIV)

Can any good come of my illness?

"It was good for me to be afflicted so that I might learn your decrees." (Psalm 119:71, NIV)

"He put a new song in my mouth, a hymn of praise to our God." (Psalm 40:3a, NIV)

"Weeping may go on all night, but joy comes with the morning." (Psalm 30:5, NLT)

"…Consecrate yourselves for tomorrow the LORD will do amazing things among you." (Joshua 3:5, NIV)

"Praise be to the God and Father of our Lord Jesus Christ, the Father of compassion and the God of all comfort, who comforts us in all our troubles, so that we can comfort those in any trouble with the comfort we ourselves have received from God." (2 Corinthians 1:3–4, NIV)

"In this you greatly rejoice, though now for a little while you may have had to suffer grief in all kinds of trials. These have come so that your faith—of greater worth than gold, which perishes even though refined by fire—may be proved genuine and may result in praise, glory and honor when Jesus Christ is revealed. Though you have not seen him, you love him; and even though you do not see him now, you believe in him and are filled with inexpressible and glorious joy, for you are receiving the goal of your faith, the salvation of your souls." (1 Peter 1:6–9, NIV)

I urge you to get into the Scriptures. Create a system that works for you, but start reading Scriptures so that you are familiar with them. I grew up memorizing verses out of context. They never meant a thing to me. We memorized things but weren't taught what they could mean to us as believers. God wants his word to mean something to us. I am a big advocate of reading Bible verses so often that they become familiar, meaningful words. God wants his word in our hearts so we won't sin. He also wants us to be well-acquainted with his precepts and nature. I urgently needed to learn of his nature. As I sought him out, I discovered his compassion and tenderness toward me. It would thrill me if you would find that in him, too.

As I fine-tuned my Scripture reading process, my prayer life remained strained. I didn't possess the words I needed to make my requests. Numerous times I would simply pray, using my index cards as a guide. I would say to God, "You talk about giving peace beyond all understanding. Could you give me that please? You say you will quiet me with your love. Can you quiet my mind today? You say you will meet all my needs. Can you help me make supper tonight?" Those were my typical prayers. In all honesty, I knew they were powerful. My heart was right, and I totally trusted God to answer my requests. I clung to the truth of Romans 8:26 (NIV), "In the same way, the Spirit helps us in our weakness. We do not know what we ought to pray for, but the Spirit himself intercedes for us with groans that words cannot express." I never before experienced that phenomenon. But I am here now to testify to that truth. My mind was so jumbled that I didn't know where to begin with my prayers. Thank God for the Holy Spirit, living in me. He knew what I needed, so he knew what to pray. He also prompted dozens of people to pray for me. There were days that I had no wits about me but I knew friends and strangers alike were praying for me.

Never underestimate the power of prayer. For years I earnestly felt prayer was a waste of time. I couldn't fathom that God cared at all about what I had to say. Then Philippians 4:6 hit me like a ton of bricks. It invites us to pray about everything instead of worrying. Many of my closest friends are worriers. I cannot grasp the agony they endure. I am grateful that I have never had that mindset. However, I must confess that I am an obsessor. I like to analyze things and play out scenarios in my mind. I enjoy thinking things to death. I love to make lists of pros and cons. I take pleasure in making lists of any kind. Somehow, it makes me feel as if I'm in control of something in my chaotic world. But let me tell you, nothing makes me feel better deep in my heart, than when I *don't* do all that stuff. When I just pray and let God do his thing, life is much better. I do believe I am strong, smart, and able to do a lot on my own. But God knows what's best for me. God has the power to do things. I don't. If I have any skills or abilities, they come directly from him. He does require us to use what he's given us. But we can't access God's power without prayer. It took me almost a lifetime to start to appreciate this concept. Early in my faith, I presumed I was supposed to pray for missionaries and sick people. In my own life, prayer didn't apply. I expected myself to be busy doing churchy things, not developing a relationship with God. I was too busy to pray. I eventually came to the realization that I didn't understand prayer at all. The following is an excerpt from *Too Busy Not to Pray* by Bill Hybels:

> Prayer is an unnatural activity. From birth we have been learning the rules of self-reliance as we strain and struggle to achieve self sufficiency. Prayer flies in the face of those deep-seated values. It is an assault on human autonomy, an indictment of independent living. To people living in the fast lane, determined to make it on their own, prayer is an embarrassing interruption...In spite of the foreignness of the activity, we pray. Why are we drawn to prayer?... We pray because, by intuition or experience, we understand that the most intimate communion with God comes only through prayer...Through prayer God gives us his peace, and that is one reason even self-sufficient people fall on their knees and pour out their hearts to him. But there is another reason. People are drawn to prayer because they know that God's power flows primarily to people who pray.[1]

God wants us to know him. He wants to give us peace. He longs to show his power through our weaknesses. God can, will, and does do the impossible when we ask him in prayer. He wants us to ask for his help. He knows we can't do all of this by ourselves. That was, perhaps, the biggest eye-opener for me. God never expected me to go through this illness alone. I prayed to him the best I could. My prayers were simple, not beautiful. They were honest and direct, not long-winded and pious. I just got on my knees and pleaded for help. I didn't even know what help I needed, but God did. Since I asked for his intervention, a truck load of help arrived! Matthew 7:11 (NKJV) says, "If you then, being evil, know how to give good gifts to your children, how much more will your Father who is in heaven give good things to those who ask Him!" I never before comprehended that God wanted good things for me. I didn't think he wanted bad things for me either. I never contemplated the fact that he concerned himself with me at all. When I think about my children and how much I love giving gifts to them, it gives me goosebumps. I look forward to Christmas, birthdays, and any other time to give them gifts. I love doing simple things for them. We enjoy getting ice cream, going swimming, taking bike rides to the park, having friends over to play. I am a faulty mother who does the best she can. If I can give these good things to my children, imagine what God, the creator of the universe, can give us? When I can give a Barbie or a Dilly Bar, God can give life. I can give my kids a day at the zoo. God can give hope. We can have a movie night with popcorn and juice boxes. God can give peace. Do you see how God's gifts are so much more precious than ours? He wants to give us good things. He came to earth so we could have more than a mediocre life; he came so we could have abundant life.

 Since I was so feeble in my attempts at prayer, I leaned

heavily on the godly women around me. God surrounded me with a wonderful group of women who prayed for me. I knew, without any doubts or questions that people were praying for me. They didn't always know what I needed, but they left that part up to God. They simply believed God would intervene in my situation if they faithfully prayed. It fascinated me to hear of people praying for me who didn't have a clue as to my circumstances. They just felt called to intercede on my behalf. Prayer is such a meaningful gift that we can give others. It is nearly impossible for me to explain the power and comfort the prayers of others have had on my life. I sensed a new warmth and depth of relationship. It sustained and refreshed me to be lifted up in prayer as others tapped into the power of God for me. What an awesome experience. In turn, I saw people open their eyes to the possibility of answered prayers. I witnessed, first hand, women believing in the reality and purpose of prayer for the first time. My ordeal actually helped some women see talking with God as important. What an honor and joy that was for me.

A life without Bible reading and prayer is a life without God. I am making you a promise. First, if you read God's word, you will be changed. You will be uplifted, supported, sustained, enriched, and strengthened. You will be pouring a firm foundation for your life. You will feel his love and understanding. There is power in the Scripture. It is useful for everything you need in life. His word will give your life direction and purpose. God wants to meet your needs and he can sure do it through his written word. If you dive in there, I guarantee you won't be wasting your time. God will deeply change your life through his word. I know because he did it with me. Second, spend time praying. Let prayer change your life! It will. God wants us to tap into his supernatural power. I Thessalonians 5:17 (NKJV) says, "Pray without ceasing." Why on earth would the Bible include that concept if it wasn't important? A life without prayer is powerless. I urge you to live your life in a disciplined manner, full of Bible study and prayer. God will give you all the direction, purpose, peace, relationship, and power you could ever need. With those elements of faith as your firm foundation, you are guaranteed to live an abundant life.

Food for thought:
"Work as if everything depended on you and pray as if everything depended on God."
—D.L. Moody, evangelist

"To be a Christian without prayer is no more possible than to be alive without breathing."
—Martin Luther, German religious reformer

"Whether we like it or not, asking is the rule of the kingdom. If you may have everything by asking in his name, and nothing without asking, I beg you to see how absolutely vital prayer is."
—Charles Spurgeon, English preacher

"Groanings which cannot be uttered are often prayers which cannot be refused."
—Charles Spurgeon

"If you are strangers to prayer you are strangers to power."

—Billy Sunday, evangelist

"In the book of life, the answers aren't in the back."

—Charlie Brown

Life After the Psych Ward

"I am still confident of this: I will see the goodness of the Lord in the land of the living." (Psalm 27:13, NIV)

I look forward to the next phase of my life's journey with much anticipation. I believe that God has taught me innumerable lessons throughout my painful illness. I'm quite anxious to get back to the land of the living and feel human again. I pray that no one would ever have to suffer from PPD to learn all that I have. Unfortunately, PPD is part of motherhood for a whole lot of us. When God said to Eve that there would be pain in childbirth, I firmly believe that PPD was included. On the flip side, I can't imagine God planned for us to have babies and then be miserable forever. That just isn't the God I know. The God who loves me might allow me to get sick, but he won't let me stay that way. He provides a way out. He wants us to come to him for healing. If we seek him, he will heal us. According to Beth Moore, in her Bible study titled *A Woman's Heart: God's Dwelling Place*, "No matter how we resist the process, healing is a cooperative effort. Often believers let their Healer extract a portion of their spiritual malignancies, then force Him to cease because of their lack of cooperation. Will you allow Him to finish the good work He began in you?"[1] I can honestly report that I am ready for him to finish this work! I sought him, and he healed me. He didn't do it half way either. I'm fully recovered and anxious to share my story with others.

I've had many people ask me questions I haven't had answers for. I've now had a full year to contemplate their questions. And, during this time of healing, I've had plenty of lessons to examine. Now that the worst is over, I want to better organize all the information I've learned. One of my favorite ways to present information is by simply answering these questions: who? what? when? where? why? and how? I will answer these for you, to testify to God's power at work in my life.

Q: *Who are the people that* PPD *impacts?*

A: I thank God, in advance, for what he's going to do as a result of my illness. I didn't suffer without purpose. I feel my purpose is to minister to those who are hurting. I sense a huge burden to teach others about postpartum depression. I feel passionate about supporting women who are suffering. There are a lot of women who suffer from postpartum depression. If that is you, my prayer is that you will be uplifted by my story. I hope that you will find solace in the Scriptures. I want you to feel the love of Christ. I hope you now realize that you are not alone. There are other women who are suffering. If you do not have postpartum depression, then there must be some special reason you are reading this. I pray that you will be better equipped to serve others who are in need. Hopefully, you gleaned some useful information. God expects you to minister to friends or relatives.

My depression had a huge impact on my life. It has also impacted my friends, neighbors, children, and husband. I pray that it will have a positive impact on other women and their families. I earnestly hope and pray that my story had an impact on you. One way or another, you were changed. Maybe you learned a thing or two. Perhaps I dispelled a few misconceptions about postpartum issues. Hopefully, you were encouraged and uplifted. I pray you saw a few Scriptures in a new light. I urge you, regardless of your situation, to spend more time in prayer, Scripture reading, and service to others. As you do these, God will transform your life. That is an investment that will bear eternal rewards.

One special group of people that must be mentioned is children, for postpartum depression deeply impacts them. Most small children don't have any understanding of what is happening. Mine believed I was sick and in pain. They had no clue that it was such a big deal. I believe that if I had not treated my depression, my family would have suffered a lot longer. But I was proactive and got help early on. There's an old saying that, "If Mama ain't happy, ain't nobody happy." If Mommy's emotional and physical health are shot, the life of the family is trampled. Children need their mothers to be well. Children need mothers who can participate in their lives.

The toll on husbands is tremendous. A husband needs his wife to be well. He counts on her to function as both wife and mother. I wasn't much of either during my illness. My husband patiently endured the ordeal while it all unfolded. I know he suffered an extraordinary amount of pain and loneliness. Depression hurts everyone in your family. It is not a good idea to avoid getting help supposedly to protect your family. I did that with my husband, and it was one of the stupidest mistakes of my life. We both paid a huge price for my pride. I'm not sure of all the ways my sickness affected my husband. I do know that he never complained while he ran the house and still worked full time. Even though he didn't verbalize his struggles, I know how exhausted he was both physically and emotionally. I think it was such an overwhelming experience that he cannot find the words to describe how it affected him. I urge you to get help. If you don't do it for yourself, do it for your husband and children. They deserve the best *you* there can be. Quite frankly, you do too.

Q: What advice can I give you?

A: I want to instill hope and courage in women who suffer with postpartum depression. I want others to know that God can get them through anything. If he did it for me, he can do it for you! But how does that translate into every day living? I have some practical tips that I am burdened to share with you. Some of these might seem obvious. However, you might need someone to give you permission to make your health a priority. It is important for me to come clean at this point. I failed to do many of the following things I now suggest, and I really paid for it. From my own experiences, I learned the hard way that my health is important.

1. Nurture yourself.

    It's okay to take care of yourself. It's actually recommended. Take bubble baths. Paint your nails—all twenty of them. Wear make-up. Get a haircut. Work on your baby's scrapbook. Read a book for fun—not a book on parenting or motherhood. Make your needs a priority. Don't waste energy on feeling guilty. You can't take good care of your child if you aren't well.

2. Sleep.

    I never slept when my third baby did. I was a total insomniac. I could not turn off my to do list that was running through my head. I was exhausted all the time. I never felt rested. Even when I was able to take naps, I either didn't or couldn't. Your body needs time to rest, especially in the early weeks. Lie down on the couch and read a magazine. Close your eyes and listen to music. Do something to rest. Your postpartum body can't go a million miles an hour, twenty-four hours a day. If you try it, you will eventually crash and burn.

3. Eat nutritiously.

    I've never been great in this department. I love chocolate, ice cream, soda, cheeseburgers, pizza, cinnamon rolls—you get the picture. I'm telling you, eating M & M's instead of lunch is a bad idea. Drinking Coke at 9:00 in the morning won't really pick you up. Eating and drinking well will be beneficial to you and your baby—maybe even to your hips!

4. Exercise moderately.
    I love to exercise. I do it because it makes my body feel alive and well. However, I must admit that postpartum exercise has never been a high priority for me. Short walks are great for both you and baby. Everyone needs fresh air, especially brand new mothers.

5. Stay in touch with friends.
    You need to be connected with your friends. Make it a priority to be in touch with other new mothers. If you can walk with friends or call them, do it. E-mail was my best friend in the early postpartum months. I couldn't talk on the phone without crying. But I could e-mail friends without trying to pull myself together. You need other women to support you; find them and be in close contact. Whatever best meets your needs, do it. Dinners, walks, exercise, shopping, Bible study, watching movies—these are all things you can do to stay connected to others.

6. Turn on your answering machine and leave it on for a while.
    I turned off my phone and just didn't care. I couldn't deal with anyone for a long time. Anyone who loves you will understand. The others? They aren't a priority and that's okay. The phone can be demanding and stressful; it's quite healthy to ignore it.

7. Your thank-you notes can wait.
    I didn't do a great job of writing thank-you notes this time around. I wrote multiple notes to the same person and left quite a few family members off the

list. I offended some people and was quite shocked by their displeasure. I'm a big believer in saying thank you for gifts I've received. However, I was so sick that I couldn't function. At the time, I didn't think writing thank-you notes was that important. I decided to quit feeling guilty that I missed a few people on my list.

I recently received an e-mail from a friend with tips for simplifying life. One of the tips dealt with thank-yous. It suggested that at baby showers, you have thank-you notes for the mother-to-be. Everyone at the party addresses a thank-you note to themselves before the end of the party. That way all the envelopes are already addressed. It would be even nicer if someone could put return addresses on the envelopes for the mother-to-be. Another suggestion? How about placing a post-it note on each card, telling what your gift was? (The crème de la crème would be if each person would write their own card and leave a space for the new mother's signature!) Thank-you notes don't have to be so stressful.

8. When someone asks what they can do to help, tell them.

Prioritize what needs to be done, and let others help you. If you need help with laundry, just say so. Pride gets in the way of our getting help. How silly. We've all been there, when the load is just too much. Don't be shy. If someone asks, surely they mean it. I don't suggest you print your to-do list and send it to all your neighbors. If there are willing hands, praise God for them.

9. Learn how to say "no."

    It took postpartum depression for me to learn this. Saying no to others is more like saying yes to myself. I know Christ wants us to be others-centered. However, when we are a mess, we need to take care of ourselves. If you get as sick as I did, you can't take care of others. I couldn't take care of my husband or children, much less my home. I put myself at the bottom of my to-do list. And I paid the consequences.

    Once I said no to some significant commitments, it became easier. I must confess that the first time was the hardest. It wasn't because I thought I was disappointing others. I wanted to earn the title of superwoman all for myself. Once I realized that there was no such award, I could say no. No one noticed that I gave myself some margins for living. I did though. I was much happier when I had some breathing room. Once I was well, I found it was still okay to prioritize myself and my family over all the "things" I could be doing.

10. Simplify everything.

    As you begin to have children, life needs to be simplified. The more children you have, the simpler it needs to be. You do not always have to be perfectly put-together, but you do need to be organized. There are two books that I highly recommend you read. *Simplify Your Life* by Marcia Ramsland is a brilliant book covering tips, systems, and habits for getting and staying organized. The back cover describes it well: "Offering practical solutions designed to change your life immediately, this simplified style of living gives you and your loved ones more time to do the things you really enjoy-starting today!" 2 *A Positive Plan for Creating More Calm, Less Stress* by Karol Ladd is possibly my favorite book of the last decade. Ladd writes, "The only person who has a stress-free day is the one who isn't breathing anymore!" 3 Once she dispels the myth that there is a perfect, stress-free home, she offers steps in a plan for creating calm instead of chaos. She explains how to develop a calm environment, refresh your spirit, renew your body, roll with the punches, and strengthen family relationships. No matter how tired you are, you must read these books. They gave me tips that changed how I dealt with everything in my house. I was refreshed and equipped to deal with real life. Better yet, these women gave me permission to be less than perfect.

Q: When has God been faithful?

God is always faithful; it's part of his nature. There will be times we don't feel God's presence. But God's presence isn't contingent on our sensing it. He won't leave us or forsake us. We are precious to him. He created us. He wants us to be complete women of faith. Life's circumstances cannot be avoided. When the storms of life hit, we only have one true rock: Christ. Our whole world can be turned upside down, but Christ isn't going anywhere. He is loyal and trustworthy; he won't leave us alone. I can attest that God didn't leave me alone during my illness. Part of the way he shows himself is through the presence and love of others. I was surrounded by friends, neighbors, and people willing to help. My entire sphere of influence gathered around me. People prayed for me, my husband, and my three children. God gave me a true sense of peace. I felt comfortable and loved even when it didn't make sense to feel that way. Who feels secure and hopeful in the middle of a crisis? With God's power and presence, a Christian can. That's one thing that will set us apart from the rest of the world. We aren't promised a light load. But Jesus does say that he'll carry our burdens for us. My load was way too heavy. He carried it for me and we made it through the storm, together.

Q: Where should you go for help?

You must contact a professional if you recognize any symptoms of postpartum depression. Untreated depression can quickly escalate into a serious situation. Call your obstetrician if at all possible, but if necessary, contact your family doctor. Get counseling from your pastor. Join a support group. Seek the help of a psychiatrist or psychologist. Read everything you can get your hands on, to support and educate yourself. Surround yourself with positive and helpful people. Get on your knees and pray to God. He will get you through this!

If you know someone with postpartum depression, urge them to seek help. Even if they get angry at you, don't let your friend or relative go untreated. Most women with postpartum issues don't get the medical attention they need. As a result, their depression lasts several months longer than necessary. If you love someone who is in pain, you may be the one who can prompt them to access professional help.

Besides all the help that is out there, there is a Healer! If I had not asked God to intervene in my situation, who knows what would've happened? I acknowledged early on that I needed help. If I had stalled in my denial or pride, I would have had a rougher time of it. Don't wait until all else fails—seek God first. He will mobilize all the help you need.

Q: Why do women have to suffer with postpartum depression?

We don't really know. It's just a fact of motherhood for a lot of people. Some women get morning sickness whereas others don't. One labor and delivery might be a piece of cake; another might be a never-ending nightmare. Some people have a smooth transition into motherhood; others do not. Some women are forced to deal with the emotional and mental roller coaster of PPD; others don't have a clue as to what it is. God made us all different. We can't accurately predict who will get PPD. All I know is that God wants us to come to him for total healing. He wants us to enjoy the precious moments we have with our newborn. He longs for us to have special bonding time with him and our baby in that first year. He is saddened if we are robbed of that. Instead of asking God, "Why me?" we should just ask for his merciful help.

Q: How is postpartum depression still misunderstood?

Just a few weeks ago, my husband and I were watching mindless television late at night. We were visually assaulted by a horrendous skit, depicting a mother suffering from PPD. She was crying uncontrollably and threw her baby (thank God it was a doll) across the room. Just that picture made my skin crawl because we do hear of similar atrocities in the news. Is that what the world thinks PPD is? Most everyone I personally know thinks postpartum depression only shows itself in a massive, psychotic way. Yes, these extreme things do happen, but they are not the norm. Less than ten percent of women exhibit as many symptoms as I did. Less than one percent exhibit psychotic behavior. Why is it, that in our culture we only hear about the one percent? We love drama. The bigger and wilder the story, the better. It boils down to the almighty dollar. Juicy stories sell books, movies, newspapers, you name it. Not too many women with PPD have juicy stories. But, they are faced with the tough reality that depression is personal and difficult. Each case is different, but the world tends to treat all depressed women the same. At www.drdonnica.com, she writes a short article called "Debunking the Myths, Misconceptions, and Misinformation About Postpartum Depression."

Here's the truth:

- PPD is a real medical disorder. It doesn't mean the woman wasn't cut out to be a mom or that she didn't want her baby.
- PPD is treatable. Moms who are treated for PPD are just as likely to become "good mothers" as those who were not affected by PPD.
- If you are given an anti-depressant, or are referred for counseling, it doesn't mean you are crazy. On the contrary, it means you are being responsible and taking care of a potentially serious medical illness.

- If you have PPD once, you may have it again (50% chance), but not necessarily. If you have it again, it may vary in severity.4

There is also a common misconception that PPD will just go away by itself. Medication is essential to leveling out the chemicals in the brain. If left untreated, the mother will most likely suffer for about a year. How cruel to let yourself suffer so long. The sooner you get treatment, the sooner you can enjoy your baby.

Another problem I've discovered is that PPD is often overlooked for many reasons. The mother or her family members might attribute her strange behavior to stress or lack of sleep. All women are tired and stressed at the start of motherhood. Women with PPD cannot cope at all with any additional stress. The brain is the most complicated organ in the body. Even the slightest chemical and hormonal changes can reek havoc on a new mom. If you question your ability to cope or you aren't sure your emotions are in check, don't disregard it. If your emotions are all over the map for more than two or three weeks, get help. Don't sweep it under the rug and chalk it all up to stress.

As I write this, it is now eleven months postpartum. I have just weaned my baby boy and had my last round of hormonal craziness. I was warned by a couple of doctors that this last hormonal shift could be the worst. I only spent one horrible night with night sweats, chills, fever, vomiting, and insomnia. I was terrified that I was going to have a rough road of it. I'm grateful that I was aware of God's presence. I knew he was with me and wasn't leaving. Lamentations 3:22–23 (NIV) says, "Because of the Lord's great love we are not consumed for his compassions never fail. They are new every morning; great is your faithfulness." I praise God, for morning did come and it was a new day. My hormones did level out, and God gave me peace. And I cling to the promise that God made in Joel 2:25, (NIV), "I will repay you for the years the locusts have eaten…" I'll have to admit, I've had the "locusts" eat up some time this year. I hold on to the hope that God will restore that time to me and my family. I pray that when I look back on this year, I will smile and remember wonderful things. I want to look back at pictures of me and my kids and have only good memories. Most of all, I want to remember this as the biggest year of my life, in that God completed our family by giving us our son. But in another way, I want to recall that this was the year God became my healer. I also know him better as my rock, shelter, counselor, strong tower, and friend. I made plans, but he established my steps. He prompted friends to pray for me. He brought me all the right doctors and counselors. He gave my husband a strength I can't find words to describe. He loved my kids when I was too sick to do so. He loved me in a way I've never felt loved before. His love lifted me out of my pit of despair. He truly was and is the lifter of my head.

Food for thought:
"It isn't the mountains ahead to climb that wear you out; it's the pebble in your shoe."

—Muhammed Ali, boxer

"It's what you learn after you know it all that counts."

—John Wooden, basketball coach

"Belief is a wise wager. Granted that faith cannot be proved, what harm will come to you if you gamble on its truth and it proves false? If you gain, you gain all; if you lose, you lose nothing. Wager, then, without hesitation, that He exists."

—Blaise Pascal, French mathematician and philosopher

"What we are seeking is excellence, not perfection. Perfection is for our own self-gratification, excellence is for the glory of God."

—Olan Hendrix, pastor and leadership trainer

"Comfort and prosperity have never enriched the world as much as adversity has."

—Billy Graham, evangelist

Listen to the MUSTN'TS, child,

Listen to the DON'TS

Listen to the SHOULDN'TS

The IMPOSSIBLES, the WON'TS

Listen to the NEVER HAVES

Then listen close to me—

Anything can happen, child,

ANYTHING can be.

—Shel Silverstein, *Where the Sidewalk Ends*

"I can do all things through Christ who strengthens me. (Phillippians 4:13, NKJV)

Endnotes

Chapter 1

1. Karen R. Kleiman, M.S.W., and Valerie D. Raskin, M.D., *This Isn't What I Expected: Overcoming Postpartum Depression* (New York: Bantam Books, 1994), 5.
2. Beth Moore, *A Woman's Heart: God's Dwelling Place* (Nashville, TN: LifeWay Press, 1995), 87.

Chapter 2

1. Karen Kleiman, M.S.W. "Postpartum Depression: When having a baby gives you more than the blues." Pregnancy Today. www.pregancytoday.com/articles/297.php?wcat=414.
2. Karen Kleiman, M.S.W. "Postpartum Depression Risk Assessment During Pregnancy." Postpartum Stress Center, www.postpartumstress.com/ppd-risk-assessment-during.html.

Chapter 6

1. "What If—So What?" http://hem.passagen.se/tildau/panic/sowhat.html.
2. "What If—So What?" http://hem.passagen.se/tildau/panic/sowhat.html.
3. Marcia Purse. About.com. www.bipolar.about.com/cs/mania/a/bl_racing.htm.
4. Max Lucado, *And the Angels Were Silent* (Portland, OR: Multnomah Press, 1992), 90.

Chapter 7
1. Stephen R. Covey, *The 7 Habits of Highly Effective People* (New York: Simon & Schuster, 1989), 81–83.
2. Beth Moore, *Believing God* (Nashville, TN: Lifeway Press, 2004), video series.

Chapter 9
1. Bill Hybels, *Too Busy Not to Pray* (Downers Grove, IL: InterVarsity Press, 1998), 9–12.

Chapter 10
1. Beth Moore, *A Woman's Heart: God's Dwelling Place* (Nashville, TN: LifeWay Press, 1995), 37.
2. Marcia Ramsland, *Simplify Your Life* (Nashville, TN: W Publishing Group, 2003), back cover.
3. Karol Ladd, *A Positive Plan for Creating More Calm, Less Stress* (Nashville, TN: LifeWay Press, 2005), vi.
4. Donnica L. Moore, MD. "Debunking the Myths, Misconceptions, and Misinformation about Postpartum Depression." www.drdonnica.com, The First Name in Women's Health. www.drdonnica.com/myths/00000393.html.